Mayo Clinic on Osteoporosis

Stephen Hodgson, M.D.

Editor in Chief

Mayo Clinic
Rochester, Minnesota

Mayo Clinic on Osteoporosis provides reliable information about osteoporosis and fractures with a focus on self-help. Much of the information comes directly from the experience of physicians, nurses, research scientists, therapists and other health care professionals at Mayo Clinic. This book supplements the advice of your personal physician, whom you should consult for individual medical problems. *Mayo Clinic on Osteoporosis* does not endorse any company or product. MAYO, MAYO CLINIC, MAYO CLINIC HEALTH INFORMATION and the Mayo triple-shield logo are marks of Mayo Foundation for Medical Education and Research.

Published by Mayo Clinic Health Information, Rochester, Minn. Distributed to the book trade by Kensington Publishing Corporation, New York, N.Y.

Photo credits: Cover photos and the photos on pages 1, 11, 14, 25, 85, 109, 129 and 149 are from PhotoDisc®; photo on page 65 courtesy of Osteometer MediTech.

Library of Congress Catalog Card Number: 2002117408

ISBN 1-893005-24-0

Printed in the United States of America

First Edition

2 3 4 5 6 7 8 9 10

About osteoporosis

Bone is living tissue in a dynamic state of renewal and change. Throughout your life, old or worn-out bone is continuously being replaced by new bone, keeping the skeleton healthy and strong. Osteoporosis affects this remodeling process by sapping bone of its mineral strength. Each year, thousands of Americans, primarily older adults, experience a sudden, unexpected bone fracture doing a routine activity. Most often, the underlying cause of this fracture is osteoporosis.

This latest book in Mayo's On-Health series, *Mayo Clinic on Osteoporosis*, provides a clear explanation of the condition and practical information on your prevention and treatment options. It includes the specifics of screening and diagnostic testing and interpreting your bone density test results. Individual chapters are devoted to nutrition, exercise, medications, good posture, recovery from a fracture and home safety, all vital elements of a comprehensive action plan.

About Mayo Clinic

Mayo Clinic evolved from the frontier practice of Dr. William Worrall Mayo and the partnership of his two sons, William J. and Charles H. Mayo, in the early 1900s. Pressed by the demands of their busy practice in Rochester, Minn., the Mayo brothers invited other physicians to join them, pioneering the private group practice of medicine. Today, with more than 2,000 physicians and scientists at its three major locations in Rochester, Minn., Jacksonville, Fla., and Scottsdale, Ariz., Mayo Clinic is dedicated to providing comprehensive diagnoses, accurate answers and effective treatments.

With this depth of medical knowledge, experience and expertise, Mayo Clinic occupies an unparalleled position as a health information resource. Since 1983, Mayo Clinic has published reliable health information for millions of consumers through award-winning newsletters, books and online services. Revenue from the publishing activities supports Mayo Clinic programs, including medical education and research.

Editorial staff

Editor in Chief
Stephen Hodgson, M.D.

Managing Editor
Kevin Kaufman

Copy Editor
Mary Duerson

Proofreading
Miranda Attlesey
Donna Hanson

Editorial Research
Anthony Cook
Deirdre Herman
Michelle Hewlett

Contributing Writers
Howard Bell
Lee Engfer
Rachel Haring

Creative Director
Daniel Brevick

Art Director
Paul Krause

Illustration and Photography
Brian Fyffe
Kent McDaniel
Michelle Papaconstandinou
Christopher Srnka
Rebecca Varga

Medical Illustration
Stephen Graepel
Michael King

Indexing
Larry Harrison

Contributing editors and reviewers

Mark Bolander, M.D.
Bart Clarke, M.D.
Darla J. Enright
Lorraine Fitzpatrick, M.D.
Christopher Frye
Daniel Hurley, M.D.
Ann Kearns, M.D.
Kurt Kennel, M.D.

Timothy Maus, M.D.
Joseph Melton, III, M.D.
Thomas Morgahan, M.D.
Jennifer K. Nelson, R.D.
Mehrsheed Sinaki, M.D.
Heinz Wahner, M.D.
Michael Whitaker, M.D.

Preface

Thirty years ago, osteoporosis was considered to be an unfortunate result of growing old. Few people gave credence to Dr. Larry Riggs' prediction that osteoporosis would become a preventable — in fact, curable — disease in his professional lifetime. But in part through the efforts of Dr. Riggs, a Mayo physician and true pioneer in osteoporosis research, his prophecy has largely become fact. Today, bone loss due to aging or as a result of other diseases and medications can usually be avoided or effectively managed. Future generations will not experience the degree of fracturing, pain and disability that have resulted from osteoporosis in the past.

Mayo Clinic on Osteoporosis emphasizes a take-charge approach to successfully managing the disease by providing detailed information and guidance on diet, exercise, medications and pain control. Attention is focused on reducing your risk of fracture and falling, alerting you to the importance of good posture and risky movements to avoid. There is also reliable information about the latest advances in medication and smart advice on how to evaluate your treatment options.

Mayo Clinic doctors who specialize in osteoporosis have reviewed each chapter to ensure that you receive the most accurate information. These doctors were assisted by Mayo specialists in physical therapy, nutrition and pain management.

We believe you'll find this book to be a practical resource for effectively managing osteoporosis. Use of the strategies described in these pages, together with the support of family and friends and the guidance of your personal physician, can offer you the best opportunity to control the disease and continue living an active and independent life.

Stephen Hodgson, M.D.
Editor in Chief

Contents

Part 2: Preventing and treating osteoporosis

Part 1

Understanding osteoporosis

Chapter 1

What is osteoporosis?

Osteoporosis is a disease that causes bones to become weak, brittle and prone to fracture. The word *osteoporosis* means "porous bones." That's an apt description of what happens to your skeleton if you have the disease. Due to a loss of bone tissue, bones that were once dense and strong may be unable to withstand the stress of even normal activity, such as bending over or twisting your torso to look behind you.

Until recently, the bone-thinning disease was considered a natural part of aging, like gray hair and wrinkles. But there's nothing natural about it. It isn't natural to lose 4 inches of height. And it certainly isn't natural to break a bone simply from coughing or giving a hug. But that's precisely what can happen if you're one of 10 million Americans — 80 percent of them women — who currently have osteoporosis, or if you're one of 18 million others who have bone density low enough to put them at high risk of osteoporosis.

The good news is that osteoporosis is as preventable and treatable as it is common. The keys to success are building a strong skeleton when you're young and slowing the rate of bone loss as you age. Even if you already have osteoporosis, good nutrition, plenty of exercise and taking prescribed medications can slow or in some cases even reverse its progression. It's never too late to do something about your bone health.

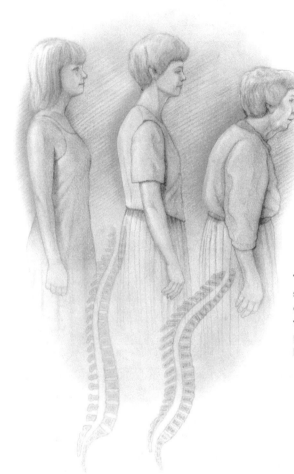

Three generations from the same family illustrate how osteoporosis can slowly lead to bone fracturing, changes in posture and gradual loss of height.

The consequences of osteoporosis

Each year osteoporosis is responsible for more than 1.5 million fractures. Typically these fractures occur in the spine, hip or wrist, but they may occur in other bones as well. A compression fracture of the spine causes your vertebrae to collapse and may lead to lost inches of height and possibly a stooped posture. Only one-third of the people who break a hip ever return to being as active as they were before the fracture. And nearly one-third go to a nursing home permanently. As if that's not enough, add chronic pain and feelings of anxiety and depression to the mix of problems that osteoporosis can cause.

Osteoporosis through the ages

Ancient Egyptian mummies with the telltale evidence of hip fractures suggest that osteoporosis has been a problem for humankind through the milleniums. But until quite recently, osteoporosis wasn't considered a disease. It was thought to be an inescapable part of aging. Stereotypes from literature, art and even television reinforced this idea. From the old woman who lived in a shoe (of nursery rhyme fame) to Granny on the television series *The Beverly Hillbillies*, old, female characters were often portrayed with a tottering walk and stooped over with the so-called dowager's hump.

In the 1830s, a French doctor studying the effects of disease on the human body observed that some people's bones were honeycombed with large holes, greatly weakening the bone structure. He was the first person to describe this condition, which he termed osteoporosis. Unfortunately, the French doctor didn't consider this to be a sign of disease and continued his investigation along different paths.

In the 1940s, Fuller Albright, M.D., of Massachusetts General Hospital, made the connection between the hormone estrogen and osteoporosis. He noticed that many of his patients who had problems with weak bones and fractures were older women past menopause. Dr. Albright believed the sharp drop in estrogen that occurs during menopause was causing the abnormal loss of bone. He correctly identified the condition as post-menopausal osteoporosis and developed the treatment that came to be known as hormone replacement therapy (HRT).

Still, even 30 years ago, the old notions prevailed. Women were told to take calcium and "live with it." Since then, new discoveries have transformed doctors' understanding. Osteoporosis is not a natural part of aging but rather a complex disease that's related to almost every aspect of your health. Osteoporosis is not just an issue for older women. It's an emerging problem among older men as well. Bone building when you're young and growing is just as important as slowing bone loss as you age.

Osteoporosis is common among postmenopausal women. If you're female and over age 50, you have an eye-opening fifty-fifty chance of breaking a bone during your remaining lifetime. Generally, your risk of breaking a hip is about the same as your combined risk of breast, uterine or ovarian cancer. Although fewer men than women get osteoporosis, men have a higher risk of death within a year of breaking a hip.

Osteoporosis is a silent disease because the bone deterioration is painless, and a bone fracture is often the first and only sign that you have the condition. Usually, by that time the disease is well developed in parts of your skeleton. But perhaps the silence is also due to a lack of knowledge. Research indicates that many people know little or nothing about the disease.

The bone bank

Think of your skeleton as a bone bank. Just as your financial health benefits from funds that you put aside and can draw on in times of need, your bone health benefits from a fund of calcium and other minerals that you store in your skeleton. Good bone health depends on keeping your bone bank account solvent, amply supplied with minerals and able to meet all of your body's needs.

Lots of daily transactions go on in your bone bank account. Throughout your life, new bone is constantly being formed and deposited. Old or worn-out bone is constantly being broken down and withdrawn. This process is how your skeleton refurbishes and maintains itself. For adults, the ideal situation is to have about as many deposits as withdrawals.

It's important to know several key terms that relate to the bone-bank concept. *Bone mass* is the total amount of bone tissue you have in your skeleton — the total assets in your account at any time. *Bone density* refers to how tightly that tissue is packed — in other words, how mineral-rich your bones are. *Bone strength* refers to the ability of bone to withstand stress, and depends on bone density, mass and quality. The more bone you have and the denser it is, the stronger your skeleton — and the stronger and deeper your bone bank account. Strong bones make it less likely that you'll develop osteoporosis or experience fractures.

Not enough bone in the bank

Generally, after about age 30, your bone bank account begins to shrink. Withdrawals from your account are exceeding deposits. You gradually begin to lose bone mass and bone density. This is normal. What's not normal is when withdrawals exceed deposits at such a rate that portions of your skeleton become weak and brittle. Scientists have yet to learn all of the reasons why this occurs.

Bone loss doesn't mean you actually lose whole bones, of course. It's the mineral content of your bones that's depleted. The outer shell of a bone becomes thinner, and the interior becomes more porous. This action bankrupts your skeleton of its strength. Under a microscope, a bone affected by osteoporosis looks like a steel bridge with many girders missing. Like a broken bridge, it may no longer be able to endure the everyday stresses and strains put on it.

Your risk of osteoporosis doesn't depend only on your current rate of bone loss. It also depends on how much bone you banked in your account when you were young and growing. That makes osteoporosis a young person's concern as much as an older adult's concern.

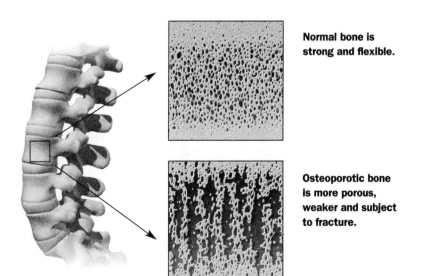

Normal bone is strong and flexible.

Osteoporotic bone is more porous, weaker and subject to fracture.

> **Osteoporosis is not osteoarthritis**
>
> Osteoporosis and osteoarthritis are different conditions with very different signs and symptoms. Osteoporosis weakens your bones. Osteoarthritis affects your joints, the places where bones are joined to one another. It wears away the cartilage that cushions your bones and keeps them from rubbing against each other. Noisy, painful and deformed joints are common signs and symptoms of osteoarthritis. Osteoporosis often goes unnoticed until a bone is broken.

Signs and symptoms

Osteoporosis is a sneak thief. Bone loss occurs painlessly over many years. Even if the bone loss is abnormally high, you probably won't experience any signs or symptoms during the early stages.

Then one day you break a bone while doing a routine task. Maybe you crack a rib while lifting a package or break a wrist after falling. At this point, osteoporosis may already be well developed and parts of your skeleton have become quite weak.

Other signs and symptoms may occur if you've experienced a compression fracture of the spine, including:

- Back pain
- Loss of height over time
- Stooped posture

It bears repeating that none of these signs and symptoms will occur because of osteoporosis unless you've had a fracture.

Having back pain doesn't necessarily mean you have osteoporosis. The most common causes of back pain are muscle strain and other conditions such as arthritis. However, back pain may be due to an osteoporosis-related fracture of the spine and its cause should be determined.

Because there are no clues to the development of osteoporosis in its early stages, it's important to be aware of the risk factors (see Chapter 4). If you become concerned, have your doctor measure your bone density before the condition weakens your skeleton. The time to act is before you break a bone.

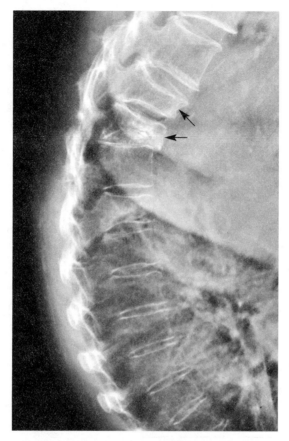

This X-ray image demonstrates how compression fractures of the vertebrae (see arrows) cause abnormal curvature of the spine and stooped posture.

Types

Osteoporosis develops for different reasons. In order to choose the correct course of treatment, your doctor will want to determine whether you have a primary or secondary form of the disease. A primary condition is the result of a specific disease process, although the direct cause is unknown. A secondary condition has a known cause, such as another disease or the use of medications. Treating that cause can often prevent future fractures.

The two most common forms of primary osteoporosis are called postmenopausal and age-related. Often, osteoporosis is a result of both. There are many secondary forms of osteoporosis, although these are less common than either primary form.

Postmenopausal osteoporosis

Postmenopausal osteoporosis happens during and after menopause as levels of the bone-building hormone estrogen decline. It's also called type 1 primary osteoporosis.

In most women, menopause occurs around age 50. Your estrogen levels begin to fall 2 to 3 years before your last menstrual cycle. The decline continues until 3 to 4 years after your last menstrual cycle. Bone loss accelerates because estrogen, which provides valuable assistance in maintaining your bone health, is no longer sufficiently available. You may lose 1 percent to 3 percent of your bone mass a year during the first 5 to 7 years after menopause. Around age 70, bone loss slows but doesn't stop. By old age, many women have lost 35 percent to 50 percent of their bone mass.

If you enter menopause with low bone mass, or if you rapidly lose bone after menopause, you're more likely to develop osteoporosis. For this reason, menopause is a good time to take steps to protect your bones, if you haven't already done so.

Age-related osteoporosis

All individuals lose bone with age. It's normal to lose between 0.4 percent and 1.8 percent of your bone mass each year up to age 80. Bone formation slows down, and bone breakdown stays the same or increases. The internal structure of your bones weakens, and the outer shell thins. These developments are a common part of aging. But it's not normal for you to lose so much bone that you develop osteoporosis.

Age-related osteoporosis is also called type 2 primary osteoporosis. In women, it's usually combined with postmenopausal osteoporosis. The aging form of osteoporosis usually starts later than the postmenopausal form, and bone loss occurs more slowly. You often don't know you have the condition until age 75 or later.

Secondary forms of osteoporosis

Secondary osteoporosis can be caused by certain diseases, surgical procedures or drugs that accelerate bone loss. Secondary causes are a factor in about 20 percent to 30 percent of postmenopausal women with osteoporosis and about 50 percent of women who are

Men get osteoporosis too

No bones about it, men also get osteoporosis. Men start to lose bone mass at a steady rate of about 1 percent a year. By age 65, men lose bone mass about as fast as women do, and by age 75 one-third of all men have osteoporosis. From this age on, osteoporosis is as common in men as it is in women.

Because many men think osteoporosis is a women's disease, they ignore simple steps they can take to prevent it. "Why worry about osteoporosis? I'm a man, right?" Don't kid yourself. One of every eight men over age 50 will have an osteoporosis-related fracture. More than 2 million American men have osteoporosis. Another 3.1 million are at risk of getting it.

approaching menopause (perimenopausal). About 50 percent of men with osteoporosis have a secondary cause.

In general, the younger you are diagnosed with osteoporosis, the more likely a secondary cause is contributing to the problem. In addition, many people who have secondary osteoporosis have or will develop primary osteoporosis as well.

For more detail about the many causes of secondary osteoporosis, see Chapter 4, which discusses your risk of osteoporosis. The chart on page 12 lists many factors that may result in secondary osteoporosis. It's not an exhaustive list, but it includes some of the more common causes.

A positive perspective on bone health

A bank account is a useful analogy to describe how your skeleton maintains itself and what happens to bones affected by osteoporosis. But the analogy shouldn't be taken too far. Low bone density — a low bank account — puts you at increased risk of osteoporosis, but it doesn't mean a fracture is a certainty in your future.

Secondary causes of osteoporosis in adults

For more information, see Chapter 4.

Medications

- Corticosteroids
- Anticonvulsants
- Excessive thyroid medication
- Certain diuretics
- Certain blood thinners
- Certain hormone inhibitors

Medical conditions

- Endocrine disorders
  » Sex hormone deficiency (hypogonadism)
  » Excess parathyroid hormone (hyperparathyroidism)
  » Cushing's syndrome
  » Type 1 diabetes
- Stomach, intestinal and liver disorders
  » Crohn's disease
  » Celiac disease
  » Primary biliary cirrhosis
  » Lactose intolerance
- Rheumatoid arthritis
- Failure to menstruate (amenorrhea)
- Prolonged bed rest due to a medical condition

Surgical procedures

- Organ transplants
- Gastric and upper intestinal surgery

Low bone mass and low bone density are good indicators of osteoporosis. However, just as your financial health can't be judged solely by what you've saved in the bank, your bone health isn't based solely on the numbers from a bone density test.

Your doctor will also need to take into consideration your bone structure, age, sex and lifestyle to determine your risk of osteoporosis. Even high risk doesn't guarantee that you'll develop the disease.

Chapter 2

The life cycle of bones

In popular imagination, bones are thought to be solid and inflexible, even lifeless. Far from being an inert frame to support your body, your skeleton has an active, if secret, life of its own. Bones are living tissue, in a dynamic state of renewal and change.

Existing bone tissue is continuously being replaced with new bone tissue in what's known as the bone-remodeling cycle. At any given moment, millions of bone-removal and bone-building projects are going on within your skeleton. This process occurs throughout your life, but the balance between how much bone is removed and how much bone is formed will vary.

Each stage of life influences developments in your bone health, starting with fetal growth in the womb and continuing through childhood and adolescence. In the young adult years, bones grow to their maximum potential in size and density. In the later years of adulthood, the process changes as you begin to lose bone more rapidly than you form it.

This knowledge of the remodeling cycle can help you understand some of the changes in your bone health and bone structure as you age. These changes vary from person to person because many factors are involved. Positive actions you can take — at any age, but the earlier the better — may help minimize negative effects of change.

Bone basics

The basic structure of bone is a fiber meshwork made primarily of the protein collagen (KOL-uh-jun). Inlaid within this framework are deposits of minerals such as calcium and phosphorus, with smaller amounts of sodium, magnesium and potassium. These minerals mix with water to form a hard, cement-like substance that makes the bone firm and strong.

Bone consists of three types of tissue: cortical bone, trabecular bone and bone marrow. Cortical (compact) bone is a dense outer shell. Its basic components are tightly packed, rod-shaped units called osteons (OS-tee-onz), which look something like long green onions bundled together. The osteons are formed from concentric

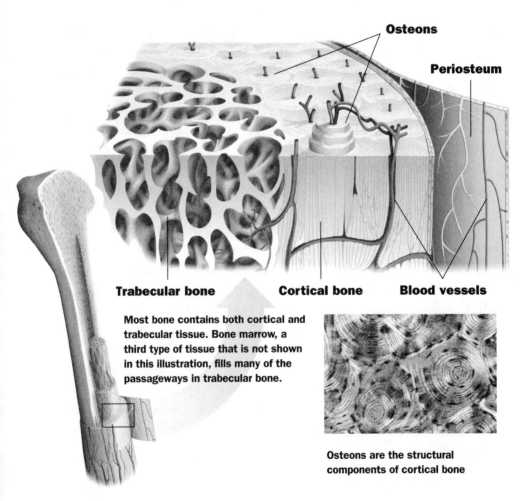

Osteons

Periosteum

Trabecular bone   **Cortical bone**   **Blood vessels**

Most bone contains both cortical and trabecular tissue. Bone marrow, a third type of tissue that is not shown in this illustration, fills many of the passageways in trabecular bone.

Osteons are the structural components of cortical bone

layers of tissue, like the layers of an onion. In each layer the collagen fibers face different directions, providing added strength.

The cortical bone surrounds a type of tissue called spongy or trabecular (truh-BEK-u-lur) bone, also referred to as cancellous bone. *Cancellous* means "lattice-like." In this type of tissue, millions of tiny interlacing strands, called trabeculae, form a complex latticework structure. The trabeculae are arranged along the lines of greatest pressure or stress in some bones.

This combination of dense cortical tissue with a supple core of trabecular tissue is what makes bones both strong and light. The skeleton is a tough but, to a certain degree, flexible structure that supports the body, protects the brain and other vital organs, and allows you to walk, run, jump, dance and move in so many ways.

Key bone builders

Minerals, like vitamins, are substances your body needs in certain amounts for normal growth and function. Because your body can't manufacture most minerals and vitamins, you must get them from the foods you eat or, in some cases, from supplements.

Minerals serve many important functions in your body, including the development and maintenance of bones. Bones also serve as a storehouse — or bank — for certain minerals, including calcium, phosphorus and magnesium. When minerals such as these are lacking in your diet, they're extracted from the reserves in your bones. Heavy withdrawals from the bone bank could impair your skeleton's ability to function normally.

Calcium is the most important mineral for bone health. Ninety-nine percent of your body's total calcium is stored in the skeleton. Besides making bones and teeth strong, calcium is needed for your heart, muscles and nerves to function properly and for your blood to clot normally.

Additional minerals that contribute to bone maintenance are phosphate and magnesium and trace amounts of a few others. Most people who eat a well-balanced diet or who take a standard multivitamin get sufficient amounts of these minerals.

Most bones contain both cortical and trabecular tissue, but the proportion of each varies from bone to bone. The long bones of the arms, legs and ribs are mostly cortical bone, whereas irregularly shaped bones, such as the pelvis or the vertebrae of the spine, are mostly trabecular bone.

Bone marrow, the third type of bone tissue, is a soft substance that fills the holes and passageways of the interior of your bones. Bone marrow manufactures your vital oxygen-carrying red blood cells and germ-fighting white blood cells. In long bones, such as the femur in the upper leg, the bone marrow fills a canal running through the central shaft.

A thin membrane called the periosteum (per-ee-OS-tee-um) covers the outer surface of a bone. This membrane contains nerves that signal pain and blood vessels that supply nutrients.

Bone remodeling

Your skeleton is a never-ending home repair project. Throughout your lifetime, bone tissue is continuously removed and replaced by new bone tissue in a process called bone remodeling (bone turnover). Although the process is imperceptible to your senses, millions of tiny sections on the surface of your bones are simultaneously under reconstruction.

Bone remodeling occurs for several important reasons. One is simply to repair damage caused by wear and tear on bones. Another is to ensure that enough calcium and other minerals circulate in the bloodstream to carry out the many bodily functions that depend on these minerals. Finally, remodeling is a response to physical activity. Your skeleton adapts to heavier loads and greater stress by forming new bone.

This skeletal regeneration occurs in two basic stages. The initial stage is bone breakdown (resorption), the second is bone formation. Each stage is carried out by a team of specialized bone cells and is regulated by hormones and other substances in the body.

During resorption, cells called osteoclasts (OS-tee-o-klasts) become active at locations on the bone surface. These cells attach themselves to the bone and, equipped with special enzymes, begin to break down the surface. As the osteoclasts eat into the bone, proteins and minerals are released and circulated in the bloodstream, sometimes for use in other parts of the body. The osteoclasts' activity forms microscopic cavities on the surface.

Bone resorption is followed by bone formation, carried out by other specialized cells called osteoblasts (OS–tee-o-blasts). The osteoblasts migrate to excavated areas and begin to fill in the cavities with collagen. This protein meshwork hardens as minerals carried in the bloodstream are redeposited in the collagen. The cycle ends when the collagen is completely mineralized — bone that was removed is now replaced.

A full cycle of bone remodeling at one site — the excavation of a cavity and the replacement of collagen and minerals in the cavity — takes about 3 to 6 months in children and adolescents and 6 to 12 months in adults. In older adults the process may take up to 18 months.

As with most remodeling projects, demolition goes faster than reconstruction. So, generally, to maintain your skeleton at any given moment, fewer sections are being broken down than are being

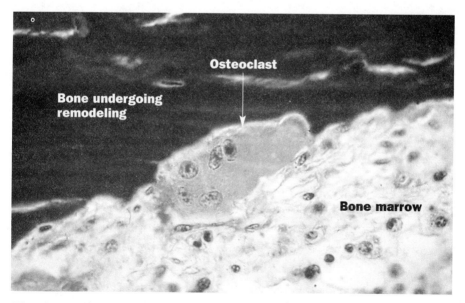

Microphotograph of a specialized bone cell, an osteoclast, breaking down the bone surface during resorption.

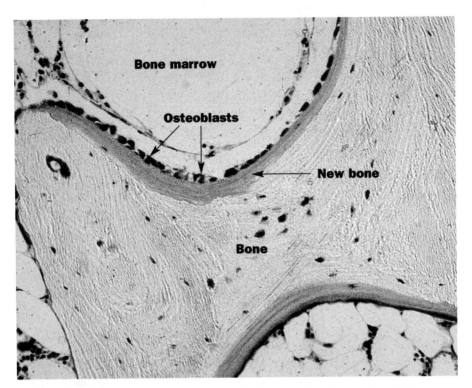

Microphotograph of bone formation showing a line of specialized bone cells called osteoblasts at work.

rebuilt. For people in their 30s, about 1 percent of the skeleton is undergoing resorption at the same time that about 4 percent is undergoing formation. At this pace the skeleton is completely regenerated every 10 years.

A carefully regulated process

The activities of osteoclasts and osteoblasts in the bone-remodeling cycle are controlled by hormones and other substances that allow bone cells to communicate with one another. Hormones also affect how much calcium is extracted from your food and how much calcium is eliminated from your body.

The word *hormone* means "to excite" or "to spur on." Hormones are chemical messengers that target specific parts of the body, to help regulate many processes and functions. Hormones are part of

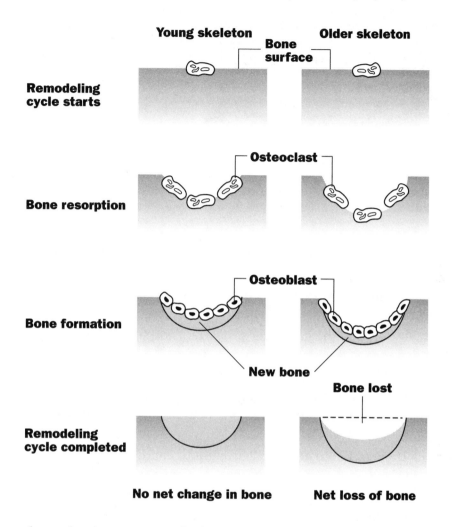

Young skeleton | Older skeleton

Bone surface

Remodeling cycle starts

Osteoclast

Bone resorption

Osteoblast

Bone formation

New bone

Bone lost

Remodeling cycle completed

No net change in bone | Net loss of bone

the endocrine system, which is a system of specialized glands. The glands produce and secrete hormones into the bloodstream as they're needed. Because the endocrine system is involved in bone remodeling, endocrinologists are among the specialists who treat osteoporosis.

The main hormone involved in bone remodeling is the parathyroid hormone (PTH), which is produced by four small glands located at the base of the neck. When the level of calcium in the bloodstream drops, the parathyroid glands secrete PTH. The hormone stimulates the osteoclasts to break down bone and release more calcium. Under special conditions, PTH can also stimulate bone formation.

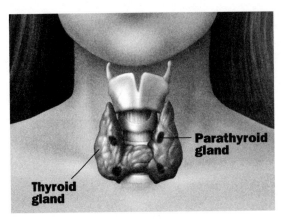

There are four parathyroid glands (indicated by the shaded areas) that lie behind the thyroid gland. The parathyroid glands produce hormones that are vital to your bone health.

Parathyroid gland

Thyroid gland

Besides PTH, other substances help regulate bone remodeling. These include calcitonin — a hormone produced by the thyroid gland — and sex hormones, such as estrogen and testosterone. PTH activates vitamin D, which is necessary to increase the amount of calcium absorbed in the gastrointestinal tract and to maintain the calcium balance in the bloodstream.

You maintain bone strength when the amount of bone that's removed by resorption is fully replaced during the formation stage. Many factors figure into this equation, including age, hormones, diet and exercise. There's great variation from person to person and from one stage of life to another. Throughout childhood, adolescence and young adulthood — the prime years of physical growth — your bone mass increases. More bone is being formed than is removed, creating a positive mineral balance in your bone bank. Changes in your body, often triggered by aging, shift the remodeling cycle from surplus bone formation or equilibrium to bone loss.

Peak bone mass

When you're young your skeleton must grow to keep pace with other developments of childhood, adolescence and young adulthood. Consequently, your bones grow larger, denser and stronger, and your bone mass increases. Following the adolescent growth spurt, young people have usually achieved up to 60 percent of their total bone mass. By age 18 skeletal growth is nearly complete.

Bone mass continues to increase slightly when you're in your 20s, and your skeleton usually reaches its maximum mass in your 30s. This is known as peak bone mass — the highest amount of bone mass that you're able to attain as a result of normal growth. At this point your bones are as fully developed in size and quality as they'll ever be.

Peak bone mass varies from one person to another. It's influenced by many factors:

- **Heredity.** Studies indicate that genetic factors account for about three-fourths of the variation in peak bone mass among groups of individuals.
- **Sex.** Peak bone mass is generally higher in men than in women.
- **Race.** Whites and people of Asian descent generally have a lower bone density than do blacks, Hispanics and American Indians.

Bone density over time

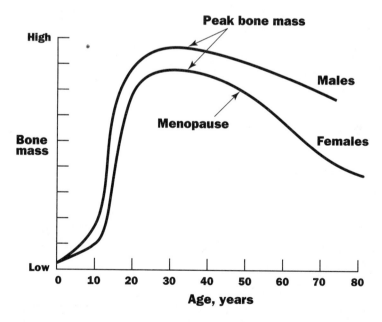

Bone density, which varies by sex and race, peaks in your mid-30s and then slowly declines with age. In general, the higher your peak bone mass, the lower your risk of having fractures due to osteoporosis later in life.

- **Diet.** People with adequate calcium and vitamin D in their diets generally reach a higher peak bone mass than do individuals who don't get enough calcium and vitamin D.
- **Physical activity.** Exercise and activity have a positive effect on your skeleton because bones respond by becoming denser and stronger.
- **Hormone production.** Estrogen, testosterone and other hormones contribute to bone formation and the maintenance of your skeleton.
- **Medical conditions.** Some chronic medical disorders and severe illnesses may reduce bone mass.
- **Lifestyle.** Smoking and alcohol abuse may have an adverse effect on bone density.

The higher your peak bone mass in your 30s, the better protected you'll be from osteoporosis, and the less likely you are to fracture in the future. That's because it takes longer for the effects of aging or illness to weaken strong bones to the point where they easily fracture. So if you're young, a great way to protect yourself from osteoporosis is to develop habits and behaviors that build bone mass. But if you're past the age of peak bone mass, don't despair. Many of these same habits and behaviors are effective in preventing or slowing bone loss.

Aging and your bones

Bone remodeling continues after you reach peak bone mass sometime in your 30s, but the balance between formation and resorption shifts. When you're young, bone formation usually exceeds bone resorption in order to meet the demands of your growing body. As you age, the rate of bone breakdown begins to overtake that of bone formation, and the number of resorption sites increases. Each year during this transition, you lose a little more bone than you gain. You'll experience about 3 percent to 5 percent of bone loss in a decade. This bone loss is universal and affects both men and women. It primarily affects trabecular bone, which is less dense than cortical bone to begin with.

Are you shrinking?

You probably reached your full adult height by about age 18 — and assumed you'd always remain that tall. Instead, as you enter middle age and beyond, you may find yourself getting shorter. How can that happen?

From day to day, no matter what your age, the disks that cushion and separate the vertebrae in your spine are being compressed during your waking hours. At night, while you rest, the disks have a chance to rehydrate and expand. You may actually be slightly taller in the morning than you are in the evening.

Over time, however, these vertebral disks naturally shrink, causing everyone to lose a little height with aging. This loss is normally slight — an inch or less. Osteoporosis can cause the vertebrae in your spine to compress or even collapse, leading to a greater loss of height than normal.

If you suspect you're "shrinking," talk to your doctor. You'll likely be screened for osteoporosis.

Osteoporotic bone

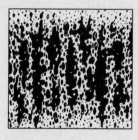

Normal bone

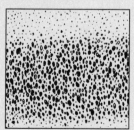

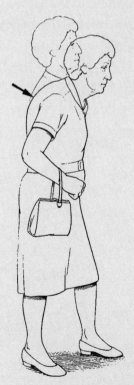

One of the possible long-term effects of osteoporosis is a series of compression fractures that can produce a stooped posture and the appearance of an upper-back hump.

The reasons for this change in the bone cycle are complex and not completely understood. With age, osteoblasts — the bone-forming cells — become less active and new bone is formed more slowly. Changes in your body's ability to absorb calcium, a decreased activity level and lower levels of certain hormones in your body also play a role. Because of these changes, your bone density decreases, and your skeleton becomes more porous and brittle.

As people get older, their intestines gradually absorb less vitamin D and calcium from the foods they eat, so less of the mineral reaches the bloodstream. The kidneys appear to lose some of their ability to conserve calcium, and as a result more calcium is lost in urine. As they age, many people eat fewer calcium-containing products such as dairy products because of intolerance to the sugar (lactose) in milk or because these products contribute to constipation.

Vitamin D production also may drop off as you age. The major source of vitamin D is sunlight, and many older adults spend less time in the sun than they once did. With age your skin also becomes less efficient at synthesizing vitamin D from the sun's rays. Older adults may consume fewer dairy products, resulting in less dietary intake of the vitamin. With less vitamin D to help in calcium absorption, the calcium that's ingested may not make it into the bloodstream.

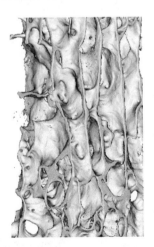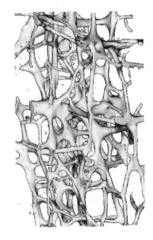

Three-dimensional images of trabecular bone from a vertebra that compares healthy bone (left) with bone that has been weakened by osteoporosis (right).

Menopause

Menopause, which normally starts around age 50, occurs when a woman's ovaries begin making less estrogen. Menstrual periods become irregular and then stop altogether. This transition may take less than 1 year or more than 2 years to complete. Declining levels of estrogen and other reproductive hormones are responsible for many of the physical and emotional changes that women may experience during this time.

Estrogen plays a variety of roles in your body. It signals your reproductive organs to mature, and it stimulates your sex drive. Estrogen also has a protective effect on bone, promoting greater density and helping regulate bone remodeling. When your ovaries produce less estrogen, bones lose the hormone's protective effect, and the rate of bone loss increases. This bone loss is irreversible, putting postmenopausal women at high risk of osteoporosis.

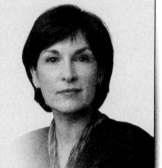

The bone loss that occurs naturally with age in both men and women is a slow process. But bone loss speeds up dramatically in women after menopause, primarily due to decreasing levels of estrogen. A woman may lose as much as 20 percent of her bone mass in the 5 to 7 years following menopause.

Men produce small amounts of estrogen, in addition to testosterone. Although men don't experience comparable bone loss at midlife, lower estrogen levels also affect men's bone density.

Around age 70 or 75, a woman's bone loss slows but doesn't stop entirely. As she grows older, she may lose 35 percent to 50 percent of her bone mass. A man may lose 20 percent to 30 percent as he ages.

Because of lower peak bone mass and accelerated bone loss following menopause, women are more likely to develop osteoporosis than men are, and their bones are more likely to fracture. Men generally have larger skeletons and more bone mass than women do, so the bone loss caused by aging is less detrimental.

Maximizing peak bone mass

Much about the bone-remodeling cycle is determined by your genes, and a certain amount of bone loss can be expected as you age. How much calcium and other minerals that have been deposited in your bone bank during the years of peak bone formation is critical. A high peak bone mass can counteract or cushion the impact of bone loss in your later years and may lower your lifetime risk of fracture. You can take many positive actions to influence the bone cycle:

- Consume a balanced diet with adequate calories, vitamins and minerals, especially calcium and vitamin D.
- Get regular exercise because physical activity contributes to higher bone mass.
- Avoid smoking and excessive alcohol use.
- For teenage females just starting to menstruate, avoid excessive dieting and other behaviors that can interfere with the timing of menstrual periods.

Even if you're past the age of peak bone mass, these actions can still help keep your bones strong and healthy. For more information, see Chapter 7.

Chapter 3

Fractures and falls

A fracture occurs when a bone can't withstand the physical force that's exerted on it. It's often the result of a fall, a sharp blow or other traumatic impact. Many people sustain one or more fractures during their lifetime.

When you were a child, a broken bone may have been painful, but then you got to wear a cool cast. You may have thought it was even cooler that everyone signed the cast and drew funny faces on it. The incident might have made for a good story later on, about that time you fell out of a tree and broke your arm. But for older adults, breaking a bone can be a serious event, resulting in complications that severely reduce their independence or may even prove fatal. For this reason, preventing fractures and falls in older adults is a major focus of doctors and other health care professionals.

A bone fracture is the clearest — and most often the only — indication of osteoporosis. Each year osteoporosis leads to 1.5 million fractures in the United States, including about 700,000 spinal fractures and 300,000 hip fractures. The loss of bone density is painless and unnoticeable in its early stages. When bone density reaches a level where osteoporosis develops, bones are weakened and less able to withstand the pressures and strains of everyday activity. Fracturing is often the result of an event that you would normally consider routine, such as lifting a bag of groceries.

Common types of osteoporotic fractures

As described in Chapter 2, as you get older — particularly with bones affected by osteoporosis — the balance in the bone remodeling cycle between bone breakdown (resorption) and bone formation changes. With aging, resorption starts to occur at a faster rate than that of formation. As a result, bone density decreases and open spaces within the bone structure widen. This contributes to a loss of bone mass in your skeleton and much lighter, weaker bones that are easier to break.

Although fractures may occur in any bone in your body, the most common fractures due to osteoporosis are of the vertebrae and the hip — bones that directly support your weight. Wrist fractures also are common. Less commonly, fractures may occur in the

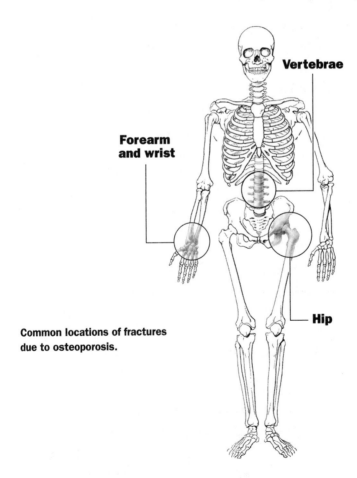

Common locations of fractures
due to osteoporosis.

pelvis and in the long bones, such as the thighbone and the humerus of the upper arm.

Spinal fractures can occur without any fall or injury — the vertebrae of your spine become weakened from daily wear and tear, leading to compression fractures. Hip and wrist fractures usually result from a fall. Hip fractures are the most serious consequence of osteoporosis. With proper rehabilitation, most people do well following surgical treatment for hip fractures. But some cases may lead to disability or death due to a serious coexisting disease.

Spinal fractures

Your vertebrae support your body, allow you to stand upright and protect the nerves of your spinal cord. The compression fractures caused by osteoporosis occur when your vertebrae lose bone density to the point of collapse. The front part of the vertebral body literally caves in. These types of fractures usually happen in the middle (thoracic) and lower (lumbar) parts of the spine. Most compression fractures occur as a result of a routine activity, such as bending over, coughing, sneezing or lifting a small parcel. If the bone density of your vertebrae is low, just one instance of this kind of activity is enough to cause a fracture. Only one out of four vertebral fractures are due to a fall.

A compression fracture often goes undetected, although sometimes it can be painful. The pain may start out with a nagging consistency or come on suddenly, and you'll likely have some tenderness around the area of the damaged vertebra. Fewer than 10 percent of people with such a fracture require admission to a hospital. Signs of multiple compression fractures include loss of height and a forward curvature of the spine. In a condition known as kyphosis (ki-FO-sis), an exaggerated curvature of the spine can give the appearance of a hump on your back.

During a physical examination, your doctor may suspect a compression fracture if you complain of sudden back pain. A spinal X-ray can more definitively reveal the compressed vertebra, which appears thinner than do normal vertebrae that adjoin it.

If a vertebral fracture isn't causing pain, treatment for the fracture itself isn't generally required. However, the underlying osteo-

Your flexible spine

Your spine is made up of 24 interlocking bones called vertebrae, which are stacked one on top of the other in a column. Each vertebra consists of the barrel-shaped vertebral body and bony projections called processes that form the vertebral arch, which protects the spinal cord. Separating the vertebrae are springy cartilage disks that act as shock absorbers, flattening under pressure to absorb the bumps and jolts of everyday life. The vertebrae are set at angles, forming four gentle curves that enhance your body's flexibility and balance.

Progressing along the spine from top to bottom, the vertebrae become larger and thicker. The seven cervical vertebrae at the top are small and delicate. They support your head. The 12 thoracic vertebrae support your arms and trunk, and the five lumbar vertebrae, which are the biggest and strongest, support the weight of most of your body and give you a stable center of gravity.

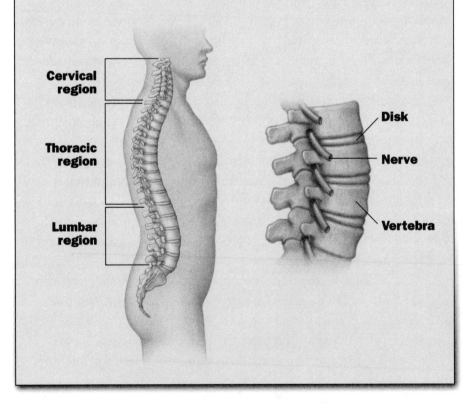

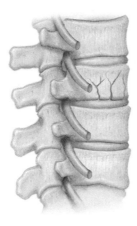

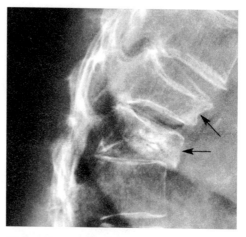

Osteoporosis may cause vertebrae to fracture and compress as a result of weakness in the bone structure.

An X-ray image of collapsed vertebrae (see arrows) demonstrates how the spine can develop an abnormal curvature.

porosis must be treated to prevent future fractures. In severe cases surgery may be an option to ease the pain or lessen the effects of extreme curvature of the spine.

Hip fractures

A hip fracture is the most serious outcome of osteoporosis. It's most often the result of a fall, especially when falling sideways or backward. Every year more than 320,000 Americans are hospitalized for a hip fracture. Doctors expect that number to grow as the American population ages.

Because older women lose bone density at a faster rate than older men do, they're two to three times as likely to experience a hip fracture. Men, however, have a higher death rate in the year following a hip fracture, mostly due to coexisting diseases and complications of fracturing. Almost a quarter of all people age 50 and older who have a hip fracture die within a year of the incident.

Ninety percent of all hip fractures occur at one of two locations along the femur, the long bone that extends from your pelvis to your knee:

- The femoral neck, a thin section of the upper femur located just below its rounded end that fits into the ball-and-socket joint of your hip

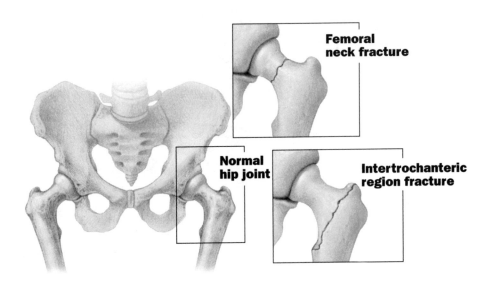

Normal hip joint

Femoral neck fracture

Intertrochanteric region fracture

Most hip fractures occur in one of two locations: the femoral neck or the intertrochanteric region.

- The intertrochanteric (in-tur-tro-kan-TER-ik) region, the part of your upper femur immediately below the femoral neck

Often your doctor can determine that you have a hip fracture based on your signs and symptoms and by observing the abnormal position of your hip and leg. An X-ray can confirm that a bone is broken and reveal exactly which part of the hip is fractured.

Although a hip fracture is usually treatable, complications from the fracture — such as a blood clot or pneumonia — can be life-threatening, particularly for older adults with other serious medical conditions such as heart disease or diabetes. If you experience a hip fracture and are immobile for a long period, you risk developing blood clots. It's possible for a blood clot to become lodged in a blood vessel in the lung, blocking blood flow to the lung tissue and causing an obstruction (embolism). This condition can be fatal if not treated promptly. Other risks of immobility due to hip fracture include bedsores and urinary tract infection.

Many older adults — including those over age 80 — do recover from a hip fracture, although the recuperation period can take up to a year, and recovery isn't always complete. During recovery many people need assistance getting around their home and doing daily tasks, such as bathing, dressing and cooking. About half the individuals over age 65 who break a hip enter a long-term-care facility while recuperating because they need assistance that's unavailable at home. Generally, the better your health and mobility before the fracture, the better your chances are for a complete recovery.

Wrist fractures

When you feel yourself falling, your natural instinct might be to extend your arms to break the impact of the fall. If the force of the fall is greater than the strength of your wrist bones, the result is often a fracture. The two main bones of your forearm are the radius and the ulna. The most common location for a wrist fracture among people with osteoporosis is at the end of the radius, just below the wrist. This type of break is called a Colles' (KOL-eez) fracture. Sometimes both bones of the forearm — the radius and the ulna — are broken by a fall.

Common signs and symptoms of a Colles' fracture include swelling, tenderness or pain in the wrist area. It's also likely that you'll find it difficult to pick up or hold anything of moderate weight. Often the wrist is deformed, inclined at an angle toward the palm of your hand. An X-ray can help your doctor determine the exact location and extent of the injury.

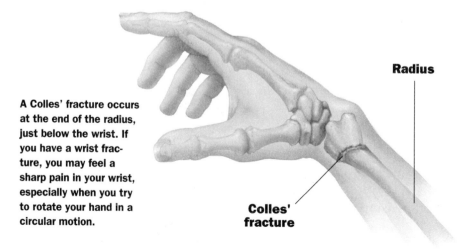

Radius

A Colles' fracture occurs at the end of the radius, just below the wrist. If you have a wrist fracture, you may feel a sharp pain in your wrist, especially when you try to rotate your hand in a circular motion.

**Colles'
fracture**

Many people recover from a Colles' fracture without problems, but older adults are at a higher risk of complications and don't always regain full mobility of their wrist joint. Possible complications include chronic pain resulting from ligament or joint damage or arthritis in the wrist. Carpal tunnel syndrome may be another long-term complication if the median nerve, which runs between the radius and the ulna, has been injured and becomes inflamed.

Risks of falling

Falling is one of the major reasons why older adults break bones. Slips and falls can happen to anyone for any reason — a loose carpet, a slick surface, a sudden surprise, an unexpected change in the pathway or dizziness caused by a reaction to medications. But as you age, falls become more common because you may be less able to react effectively to the situation. Various changes associated with aging — such as problems with balance, loss of muscle mass and

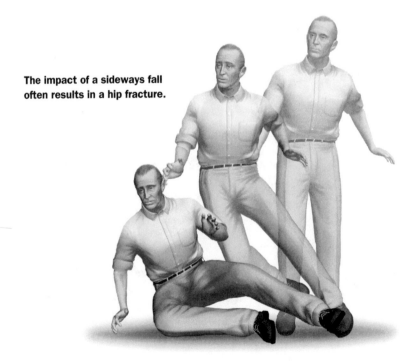

The impact of a sideways fall often results in a hip fracture.

The mechanics of a fracture

Some osteoporosis research has used engineering principles to calculate the risk of fracture. The amount of force applied to the hip or the spine by certain activities or actions is compared with the maximum amount of pressure these bones can bear — similar to calculating the tonnage a bridge can bear. Researchers were able to identify several activities and actions that involve a high risk of fracture.

One of the most significant risk factors for a hip fracture is falling sideways, either while walking or from a standing position. The impact often exceeds the capacity of an average older adult's hip to sustain the fall, resulting in a fracture. Other factors also influence the risk of fracture. For example, absorbing some of the energy of the fall with your leg muscles or using an outstretched hand to break the fall can reduce the impact on your hip. Skin and fat around the area of impact or wearing hip pads also can reduce damage caused by the fall.

The risk of a compression fracture in the spine has also been measured. By bending over at a 30-degree angle and lifting a weight of approximately 17 pounds (8 kilograms) — which can be the equivalent of lifting a small child or a bag of groceries — you can more than double your risk of a compression fracture if your bone density is low.

poor vision — can contribute to slower reaction times. Older adults also lose some of their bone strength and fatty cushioning, particularly around the pelvis, which help to break falls. In addition, they're more likely to have chronic conditions that impede their ability to move about, and they're often the ones who take medications that may cause dizziness.

About a third of people over age 70 fall at least one time each year. Although only 3 percent to 6 percent of these falls result in a fracture, the occurrence of the fracture can greatly reduce the quality of life. That's why it's so important to prevent falls. Here's a closer look at some of the main risk factors for falling, including some that you can influence or control.

Problems with balance

As you age your sense of balance declines and your reaction time slows, increasing the likelihood of falling. Under normal circumstances, balance is controlled by the signals sent to your brain from three sensory systems in your body:

- **Inner ear.** The slightest movement of your head activates sensors in your inner ear. These sensors send electrical signals to the brain, which is constantly monitoring the position of your head relative to the ground.
- **Eyes.** Visual signals help you determine where your body is within the environment.
- **Sensory nerves.** Nerves in your skin, muscles and joints send messages to your brain about the movement of your body.

Good balance depends on at least two of these systems working well. For instance, closing your eyes while washing your hair in the shower doesn't mean you'll lose your balance — signals from your inner ear and sensory nerves help keep you upright.

If your central nervous system is slow to process these signals, if the messages are contradictory or if your sensory systems aren't functioning properly, your balance may suffer. This may make it harder for you to avoid something in your path or adjust to a sudden change in the ground surface, leading to a fall. Some older adults have increased body sway while standing still, which also may increase the risk of falling.

Muscle weakness

As you get older, your muscles lose some of their bulk and begin to weaken. With time, your ligaments and tendons, the body's connective tissues, lose their elasticity and cause your muscles and joints to stiffen. Lack of physical activity also can decrease muscle mass and strength.

Combined with the changes in balance brought on by aging, muscle weakness can turn a stumble into a fall. When your brain receives a signal that you've lost your balance, it triggers your muscles to try and compensate. But if your reaction is slow and your muscles are weak, your body may be unable to maintain itself upright.

Vision problems

Much like the tissue of your ligaments and tendons, the tissue of the lenses of your eyes become less elastic with age. Less elasticity makes it harder to focus a sharp image on your retina and to see close objects clearly. Problems with seeing or changes in your depth perception make it easier for you to trip or stumble off a step.

Many age-related vision problems can be corrected with the right glasses, and older adults may find it necessary to wear bifocals or trifocals. But shifting your eyes between different focal powers in a lens can disorient you momentarily, affecting your balance and possibly causing a fall. Focusing straight ahead and lowering your head can help avoid this.

Eye conditions such as cataracts, glaucoma and macular degeneration also can affect your perception or make it difficult to see obstacles.

Chronic medical conditions

As you get older, you become more susceptible to various chronic problems that may increase your chances of falling. Conditions that affect your nervous system, such as stroke, Parkinson's disease and multiple sclerosis, may affect your balance and coordination. Disorders affecting your feet and legs, such as arthritis and peripheral nerve damage, may disrupt your ability to walk.

Chronic diseases such as emphysema or congestive heart failure may make it difficult to get around, resulting in physical inactivity and loss of muscle strength and balance.

People with decreased mental alertness, such as that caused by dementia or depression, are at increased risk of falling. In addition, flu, low blood pressure or dehydration can cause dizziness.

Reaction to medications

Some drugs may affect your balance and cause dizziness. These include certain blood pressure medications, sedatives, tranquilizers, antidepressants, cold and allergy medications (antihistamines), pain relievers and sleep medications. Other side effects from these medications may include muscle weakness, shakiness and blurred vision, any of which can lead to a fall.

Some of these medications, particularly blood pressure medications, tranquilizers and antidepressants, may cause a sudden drop in blood pressure if you stand up quickly, leading to lightheadedness or fainting. Getting up slowly from a sitting or lying position helps to prevent this sudden drop in blood pressure.

Always ask your doctor about the side effects of medications you're taking and how you might reduce these side effects. Your doctor may be able to prescribe a different drug.

Environmental hazards

Besides factors *within* your body that may lead to a fall, plenty of factors *outside* your body can cause a tumble. Although you may think that home is the safest place to be, according to the American Academy of Orthopaedic Surgeons, most falls and resulting fractures occur at home. Some potential hazards within your house include loose rugs, cluttered floors, poor lighting, exposed electrical or telephone cords, and stairs with no handrails. Walking around the house in socks or standing on something other than a sturdy step stool to help you reach for objects also can spell trouble. Any of these hazards could cause you to fall, often onto furniture, which increases your chance of a fracture. For information on making your home a safer place, see Chapter 13, which also offers tips on preventing falls outside the home.

Risks of a second fracture

Most doctors regard fractures caused by routine activities — activities that normally wouldn't be traumatic enough to break a bone — as strong evidence of osteoporosis. This kind of fracture is known as a low-trauma fracture. Compression fractures of the spine, which may result in you losing height, can occur simply from bending too far forward. This kind of fracture is often caused by osteoporosis and all too frequently goes unnoticed until the disease is well developed and your vertebrae are considerably weakened.

A low-trauma fracture not only indicates osteoporosis but also increases your risk of future fractures. Statistical records show that once you've had one fracture, your chances of another fracture are even greater. For example, the lifetime risk of a fracture of the hip, spine or wrist is 40 percent in white females age 50 and older, and almost 15 percent in white males age 50 and older. However, the risk of another osteoporotic fracture almost doubles once you experience your first fracture.

More specifically, records indicate that having a single vertebral fracture, even with no symptoms, increases your chances of subsequent fractures by at least four times, independent of your bone density. The risk of hip fracture is more than double following an initial fracture of the hip or spine. Risk of hip fracture is also increased following the fracture of a forearm or an upper arm bone.

According to guidelines published by the American Association of Clinical Endocrinologists, the two most important risk factors for osteoporosis-related fractures are (1) low bone density and (2) a previous low-trauma fracture in an adult at age 40 or older. The first factor is closely related to osteoporosis and probably doesn't surprise anyone. This may not be the case for the second factor. It implies a bone fragility and susceptibility to fracture that's too complex to be measured.

If you fracture a bone, is there something you can do to reduce your chances of a future fracture?

First, find out if your bones are thinning and to what extent you're losing bone mass. It's important to consider getting tested after breaking any bone. According to the World Health Organization, any woman experiencing a wrist fracture after menopause has sufficient cause to evaluate her bone density for osteoporosis. The National Osteoporosis Foundation recommends bone density testing for all postmenopausal women following a fracture. Some doctors recommend initial screening using the less expensive tests, and then scheduling more thorough testing as warranted.

Additional testing may also be necessary to check hormone levels and other indicators that may affect your bone health. These tests may include blood tests to check calcium and phosphate levels, thyroid function and liver function. Urine tests also may be done. For more information on these procedures, see Chapter 5.

If your bone density is low, find out what's causing the problem — whether it's osteoporosis or some other condition that's leaching minerals from your bones. Appropriate measures can be taken to increase bone density and strengthen your bones and muscles. With proper treatment of any potential underlying condition after a first fracture, the risk of a second fracture may eventually return to normal. And regardless of the results of your bone density test, they provide a benchmark for subsequent changes in your bone health.

The critical role of fracture prevention

Fractures can be life-changing events, particularly for older adults. Even a single fracture can put you at greater risk of more fractures, potentially creating a downward spiral in your health.

If you have osteoporosis but never experience a fracture, there will typically be no serious consequences of the condition. That's why it's so important to avoid breaking a bone. You can do this by treating your osteoporosis, preventing falls, practicing safe movements and activities, and not lifting more than the bones in your spine can bear. Subsequent chapters provide more information on protecting your bones. In the end, remember that it's much easier and less expensive to prevent a fracture than it is to treat a fracture.

Chapter 4

Can you reduce your risk of osteoporosis?

No one can say for sure whether you'll get osteoporosis. The disease is too complex for that. But doctors do know what makes some people more likely than others to get it. There are things about you and your lifestyle that may make you more susceptible. So it's important to be aware of the risk factors for osteoporosis and what you can take to reduce some of them.

If you already have osteoporosis, bone loss has seriously weakened your skeleton. But if you never have a fracture, you avoid the most serious consequence of osteoporosis. Pain is normally not associated with this disease unless fracturing has occurred. Even individuals with very low bone density can continue to lead active, independent lives and participate in activities they enjoy, as long as they don't break a bone.

Generally speaking, your risk of osteoporosis and fracturing depends on your bone health — the size and strength of your bones and the condition of your bone tissue. Bone health is a result of how well your skeleton developed during childhood and early adulthood and how much bone was present at the time of your peak bone mass, usually between the ages of 30 and 40. Bone health is also affected by how rapidly you lose bone mass as you get older.

Many unique factors about you have put an individual stamp on your bone health. These include family history, heredity, hormones, the quality of your nutrition, the amount of exercise you undertake, behaviors and habits in your lifestyle, and the overall state of your health. The factors that lower your peak bone mass or accelerate bone loss increase your susceptibility to osteoporosis. They are called risk factors. By taking precautions, having realistic expectations of what you can or can't do and doing everything you can to build or maintain bone mass, you may lower your risk of osteoporosis and fracture.

Assessing your chances

If you were to characterize the person most likely to get osteoporosis, you might describe a tall, thin, postmenopausal white woman who smokes, abuses alcohol, eats poorly, doesn't exercise and takes medications such as corticosteroids. Also, her mother would have had stooped posture from multiple compression fractures of the spine. But keep in mind, even if you share some of these characteristics, you're not destined to get osteoporosis. And if you do get osteoporosis, you're not necessarily going to break a bone. Conversely, some people with no known risk factors can develop osteoporosis and break their hip.

If some of the risk factors described below apply to you, discuss them with your doctor. You and your doctor can work together to prepare a prevention strategy that is both practical and achievable. If you're a woman, you may consider making these plans before you reach menopause. Even if you're past menopause, you can still take positive steps to slow bone loss.

Risk factors you can't change

Some risk factors you can't control. You were born with them or you inherited them from your parents, or they're simply an inherent part of living. But you can take measures that prevent or slow osteoporosis from developing, and you can monitor your bone health to detect abnormal bone loss as early as possible.

Sex

Eighty percent of all Americans with osteoporosis are women. Women usually reach a lower peak bone mass than men do because their skeletons often are smaller. Women also tend to live longer. So, in effect, women have less bone to lose and more time in which to lose it. In addition, when menopause occurs women experience a drop in their estrogen levels, a drop that accelerates bone loss.

Young male adults generally have 25 percent more bone mass in their vertebrae than females of similar age have. Bone mass of the male hipbone tends to be 8 percent to 18 percent greater than that of the female hipbone.

Women are three times as likely as men to break a bone because of osteoporosis. Certainly the lower level of estrogen following menopause is a major factor. Fracturing generally starts at a younger age in women than in men. Young women are four times as likely as young men to break a hip, although later in life the odds even out.

Age

The older you are — male or female — the more likely you are to get osteoporosis and the more likely you are to break a bone because of it. Fifty percent of women in their 80s have osteoporosis. For more information on how aging affects your bone health, see Chapter 1.

Heredity

Family history is a strong predictor of low bone mass, but it's not a very good predictor of your chances of fracturing due to osteoporosis. Studies show that genetic factors account for many differences in bone size, bone mass and bone density among individuals. If your mother, sister, grandmother or aunt has osteoporosis, you're more likely to get it. Research also shows that if you're a woman whose mother broke her hip, you're twice as likely to break a hip, compared with the general population of women.

Several genes affect your risk of osteoporosis. They play a role in how high a peak bone mass you'll achieve when you're young and how rapidly you'll lose bone mass later in life. You also have genes that determine when you go through menopause and genes that regulate hormones and growth factors, all of which influence bone formation and bone breakdown. Other genes affect how your body uses calcium and vitamin D or makes the protein collagen, which is an essential ingredient of bone.

But genes don't necessarily determine your bone destiny. Just because your mother got osteoporosis doesn't mean you will. By doing the right things to lower your risk, you may avoid that fate.

Race

Whites and Asians have the highest risk of osteoporosis. White women past menopause experience almost 75 percent of all hip fractures. Blacks have the lowest risk of osteoporosis, and Hispanics and American Indians appear to have an intermediate risk. The various levels of risk are based in part on racial differences in bone mass and bone density. And some Asian women, for example, tend to have a lower calcium intake in their diet. However, regardless of race, any woman who had her ovaries removed at an early age has greatly increased her risk of getting osteoporosis.

Body size

Petite women with a thinly boned frame are at greater risk of osteoporosis. They may reach a fracture-prone stage earlier because they have less bone to begin with.

Exposure to estrogen or testosterone

The greater your exposure to estrogen over your lifetime, the lower your risk of osteoporosis. Women who began menstruating after age 16 don't have the bone-building effects of estrogen for as many years as those who started menstruating earlier. Likewise, women who reach menopause early — either naturally in their late 40s or due to surgery before age 45 — lose the bone-building benefits of estrogen much earlier.

In men, a delayed onset of puberty after age 16 can shorten their lifetime exposure to the bone-building hormone testosterone and lower their peak bone mass. A low testosterone level during adult years can accelerate bone loss.

Risk factors you may influence

Certain risk factors for osteoporosis and fracturing may be more than a matter of simply having them or not having them. If one of these factors is present, your individual circumstances or certain decisions you make may modify that risk. Many forms of secondary osteoporosis are treatable, or they may occur only for a certain period of time. In many cases, you may be able to take preventive steps that compensate for increased risk.

Childbearing

Pregnancy builds stronger bones in women by raising their estrogen levels and increasing their weight. Both factors are beneficial to bone mass. Whatever your circumstances, the fact that you have one or more children or no children may be considered when assessing your risk of osteoporosis.

During pregnancy, you're sharing your supply of calcium. Breast-feeding also can drain calcium from your body, but your intestinal tract and kidneys compensate for this extra demand by absorbing and conserving more calcium. Still, if you're expecting a child, talk with your doctor about getting sufficient calcium.

Medications

Certain medications are known to accelerate bone loss and thus increase your risk of osteoporosis. These medicines may cause a form of secondary osteoporosis, or they may aggravate the kind of osteoporosis caused by aging or menopause.

Corticosteroid medicines. Long-term use of corticosteroids, such as prednisone (Deltasone, Sterapred), cortisone (Cortone Acetate), prednisolone (Prelone) and dexamethasone (Decadron), is especially damaging to bone. These medications, also called glucocorticoids, are commonly used to treat asthma, rheumatoid arthritis and other inflammatory conditions. They lower bone mass by decreasing your blood levels of estrogen and testosterone and by slowing bone formation.

Any dosage of a corticosteroid increases your risk of fracture. But these drugs have benefits. If your doctor has you taking one of these medications, he or she has good reasons for doing so. Don't stop taking it, and don't change your dose without first talking to your doctor. If you take the medicine for more than a few weeks, it's likely that your doctor will monitor your bone density and recommend drugs that prevent this type of bone loss.

Anticonvulsants. Drugs used to control seizures include phenobarbital, phenytoin (Dilantin) and carbamazepine (Carbatrol, Tegretol). If this type of medication is used over a long period of time, your liver starts to convert vitamin D in a way that causes a vitamin D deficiency. If you take one of these medications, your doctor may recommend vitamin D and calcium supplements.

Thyroid medicine. If used in excessive quantities, thyroid medications such as levothyroxine (Levothroid, Levoxyl, Synthroid) can cause hyperthyroidism, leading to accelerated bone loss. Because your requirements for the thyroid hormone can change over time, a blood test called a thyroid-stimulating hormone (TSH) test should be done annually. The test easily determines if you're taking the right amount of thyroid medicine, and the dose can be adjusted if necessary.

Diuretics. Diuretics are drugs that prevent fluid buildup in your body. In so doing, certain diuretics may also cause your kidneys to excrete too much calcium. If you're not getting enough calcium and other bone-building minerals in your diet, you may experience bone loss. The diuretics that cause this concern include furosemide (Lasix), bumetanide (Bumex), ethacrynic acid (Edecrin) and torsemide (Demadex). Other diuretics, called thiazides, may actually help your body retain calcium. Always talk to your doctor about any risks associated with your medications. You may be able to switch to a diuretic that doesn't cause a loss of calcium.

Other medications. Blood thinners such as heparin are prescribed to prevent blood clots from developing in your veins and arteries. They may cause bone loss if used over long periods of time. You may be able to switch to more bone-friendly warfarin (Coumadin).

Gonadotropin-releasing hormone agonists are a class of drugs used to suppress blood levels of estrogen and testosterone. They include leuprolide acetate (Lupron) and nafarelin (Synarel). These drugs are effective in treating conditions such as endometriosis, severe premenstrual syndrome (PMS) and prostate cancer. Reduced levels of the sex hormones can also result in rapid bone loss. Levels usually return to normal after the dosage is stopped.

Medical conditions

Certain medical conditions can increase your risk of osteoporosis by slowing bone formation or speeding up bone resorption. Some of these conditions may cause a form of secondary osteoporosis.

Endocrine disorders. The endocrine system produces hormones that help regulate many body activities. Problems with endocrine glands associated with bone growth and maintenance can disrupt your bone-remodeling cycle.

Hypogonadism occurs from a lack of estrogen and testosterone, leading to abnormal bone loss. Many factors can affect hormone production, including certain medications, various diseases of the ovaries or testes, natural aging, and eating disorders that disrupt menstruation.

Hyperparathyroidism is the result of overactive glands supplying too much parathyroid hormone (PTH) to your bloodstream. Too much PTH may release too much calcium from your bones and increase your risk of fracture.

Cushing's syndrome occurs when the adrenal glands produce too much cortisol, a corticosteroid that slows bone formation and can increase bone resorption.

Type 1 diabetes (formerly called juvenile or insulin-dependent diabetes) is associated with bone loss, especially if the condition is poorly controlled. Individuals with this condition often have a low bone mass. Type 2 diabetes (formerly called adult-onset or noninsulin-dependent diabetes) isn't associated with osteoporosis.

Disorders of the stomach, intestine and liver. Some gastrointestinal diseases can affect the bone remodeling cycle and lead to bone loss. They do so by interfering with the way your intestines absorb calcium from the food you eat and by lowering your vitamin D level.

Disorders of the small intestine such as Crohn's disease and celiac disease can result in reduced bone mass. Sometimes they're treated with a corticosteroid, which further inhibits calcium absorption and vitamin D levels.

Certain disorders of the liver are rare but notorious for causing osteoporosis. Primary biliary cirrhosis occurs when tiny bile ducts in the liver become inflamed. This disorder occurs most often among women between the ages of 35 and 60.

Lactose intolerance causes gas, stomach cramps and diarrhea when you drink milk. If you're lactose intolerant or don't eat dairy products for other reasons, it's important to take calcium supplements or to eat plenty of nondairy foods high in calcium.

Rheumatoid arthritis. This arthritic condition is an autoimmune disease, which happens when your own immune system attacks your body. The principal area of attack of rheumatoid arthritis is the lining of your joints, leading to the gradual destruction of cartilage, bone, tendons and ligaments in the joint. This disabling condition prevents people from being physically active, increasing their risk of bone loss. Rheumatoid arthritis is treated sometimes with corticosteroids and other medications that can damage bone.

Amenorrhea. Absent or irregular menstrual cycles in women of childbearing age may be a sign of low estrogen levels. This condition may be caused by eating disorders, excessive exercise or disorders of the ovaries or pituitary gland. If you have a history of abnormal menstrual cycles, your risk of osteoporosis is increased.

Surgical procedures

Organ transplants can result in bone loss because the immunosuppressant medications you must take will interfere with bone formation. You may need to take corticosteroids, which damage bone.

Gastric surgery that removes part of your stomach because of cancer or ulcers can cause bone loss because you're less able to absorb calcium and vitamin D from your food. Intestinal bypass surgery may result in abnormal bone loss years after surgery.

Prolonged bed rest

If you're on prolonged bed rest or immobilized because of stroke, fracture, surgery, quadriplegia or paraplegia, consult your doctor regarding what you can do to prevent abnormal bone loss.

Risk factors you can change

You can control some risk factors. That means you may be able to eliminate them or at least greatly reduce their effect on your skeleton. Osteoporosis is easier to prevent than to treat, and that's why these factors are so important for you to know about.

Calcium and vitamin D in your diet

Calcium and vitamin D are crucial for building strong bones and keeping them strong as you age. Not eating enough food high in calcium when you're young lowers your peak bone mass and increases your fracture risk later in life. Lack of vitamin D inhibits your ability to absorb calcium from the food you eat. Clinical studies show that supplements containing calcium or calcium with vitamin D can reduce fracture rates by about 30 percent to 50 percent in people who don't get enough of these nutrients in their diet. For the recommended amounts of calcium and vitamin D in your diet, see pages 91 and 94.

Excessive weight loss and dieting

In our weight-obsessed society, you may try to stay thin by keeping food off your plate. But if you starve your body, you starve your bones. Serious eating disorders such as anorexia nervosa and bulimia can damage the skeleton by depriving your body of essential nutrients needed for bone building.

Anorexia nervosa is an eating disorder triggered by an overwhelming fear of weight gain. It primarily affects young women. The disorder disrupts the menstrual cycle, lowers estrogen levels and, during this important time of skeletal development, inhibits a high peak bone mass. Someone with anorexia may start losing bone at an earlier age and have less bone than she can afford to lose in the first place. As many as 50 percent of women with anorexia have low bone density in their lower spine.

Excessive dieting also can harm your bone health. When you're a young adult, body weight influences your peak bone mass. Thin women tend to have less bone-building estrogen, and heavier women tend to have more. Fat cells help produce estrogen. So women who lose lots of weight through dieting sometimes lose bone mass along with the pounds. That doesn't mean you should be overweight — a condition that has other health problems associated with it — but you should try to stay within a normal weight range for your age and height.

Physical activity

Use your bones or lose your bones. Regular activity and exercise are keys to preventing osteoporosis and fractures. Children who are the most physically active often have a high bone density and reach a higher peak bone mass than do children who don't exercise enough. Lack of exercise accelerates bone loss when you're older. Studies show that adults who sit all day at a desk job and don't exercise are more apt to lose bone mass and suffer fractures than are adults who fit some activity into their day.

Weight-bearing exercise such as walking can increase or at least maintain your bone density at any age. For more information on appropriate activities and exercise that you can participate in, see Chapter 9.

Smoking

You already have plenty of good reasons to stop smoking. Here's another — smoking is bad to the bone. Smoking interferes with production of estrogen and testosterone. Smoking also disrupts calcium absorption and the bone formation part of the remodeling cycle. That may be a reason smokers — both male and female — are more apt to get osteoporosis and to have bone fractures.

Menopause, which accelerates bone loss, happens on an average of 2 years earlier in smokers than in nonsmokers. And post-menopausal smokers lose bone at a faster rate than post-menopausal nonsmokers do. Though hormone replacement therapy (HRT) protected nonsmoking women from fractures, it didn't do nearly as good a job of protecting women who smoke. Smokers tend to drink more alcohol and to not exercise or eat as well as nonsmokers. These behaviors increase your risk of osteoporosis. The good news is, if you stop smoking, even later in life, you can slow bone loss.

Alcohol use

Drinking alcohol in excess over a long period of time can increase your risk of osteoporosis and fractures. Alcohol is toxic to bone-building osteoblasts. Meanwhile, bone-removing osteoclasts may be stimulated by alcohol, increasing bone loss. Chronic heavy drinking also lowers levels of estrogen and testosterone. More than 1 ounce of alcohol a day for women and 2 ounces a day for men can begin to cause these effects.

Even moderate drinking can thin the more porous trabecular bone of your vertebrae. Although vertebral fractures are uncommon in most people younger than 50, they're much more common among those who are heavy drinkers. Furthermore, alcohol abusers are more likely to have poor nutrition and to not exercise, both of which slow bone formation. These individuals are also more likely to fall and break a bone because alcohol impairs their balance. Many individuals who stop drinking alcohol usually recover their regular bone-building abilities and, if they're relatively young, may even recover some lost bone mass.

What you can do

Osteoporosis is a treatable disease. And the fracturing associated with it isn't inevitable. You can take effective measures to maintain strong bones and a healthy skeleton. Preventing fractures is an important element of bone maintenance because the first low-trauma fracture greatly increases your risk of future fractures.

Now that you've had a chance to review the factors that can increase or decrease your risk of osteoporosis and fracturing, you may wish to discuss them with your doctor. Together you can determine whether you're at high, moderate or low risk. Generally, being at high risk means you have two or more risk factors.

Then you and your doctor can plan your strategy for lowering and even eliminating some of those risks. The earlier in life you do this, the better. But remember that it's never too late to start. You may wish to ask your doctor about a bone density test. You can learn all about this important test in the next chapter.

Risk evaluation for osteoporosis

Answering these questions can help you evaluate your risk of osteoporosis. The more yes answers you have, the higher your risk.

	Yes	No
• Are you female?	☐	☒
• Have you stopped menstruating?	☐	☒
• Have you ever broken a bone?	☐	☒
• Have you experienced a loss of height?	☒	☐
• Do you have a family history of osteoporosis?	☐	☐
• Are you white or Asian?	☒	☐
• Are you petite or smallboned?	☒	☐
• Did you start menstruation at age 16 or older?	☐	☐
• Did you have irregular periods before menopause?	☐	☐
• Were you never pregnant?	☐	☐
• Did you go through natural menopause before age 45?	☐	☐
• Were your ovaries removed before age 40?	☐	☐
• Have you taken medication for a year or more that could increase bone loss?	☐	☐
• Have you ever had a medical condition that's known to increase your risk of osteoporosis?	☐	☐
• Do you include little or no foods containing calcium in your diet?	☐	☐
• Have you dieted frequently or ever lost an excessive amount of weight?	☐	☐
• Do you not exercise?	☐	☐
• Do you smoke tobacco products?	☐	☐
• Do you drink more than 2 ounces of alcohol each day?	☐	☐

Chapter 5

Screening and diagnosis

"How do I know if my bones are weak? Do I already have osteoporosis?" These are questions you may want answered, and the sooner you get answers, the better. The sooner you can start on prevention, the better your chances of keeping your skeleton healthy. If you already have osteoporosis, the earlier you treat it, the better your chances of slowing bone loss and stabilizing your condition.

It used to be that the only way to detect osteoporosis was when you broke a bone. By then, parts of your skeleton would already be quite weak. Things are different now. A bone density test, also known as bone densitometry, can determine if you have osteoporosis before any bones are broken. It can also tell if your bone density is low enough to put you at risk of osteoporosis. This risk level is known as osteopenia (os-te-o-PE-ne-uh).

A doctor can also learn much about your bone health from giving you a thorough physical examination. This evaluation may occur before or after bone density testing. The examination is one of the best ways to identify secondary causes of osteoporosis.

After evaluating the test results and conducting a complete physical exam, your doctor can provide you with clear answers to questions about your bone health. This chapter and the next describe bone density tests in detail.

Screening vs. diagnosing

Before getting to the details of bone density testing, it's important that you're clear on the distinction between the terms *screening* and *diagnosing*.

Screening tests

Screening refers to testing someone who has no apparent signs or symptoms of a disease. If the test result registers as abnormal, it may reveal the presence of a previously unsuspected problem. Sometimes, screening tests are less sensitive, but also less expensive, than diagnostic tests. You'll generally undergo a screening test for osteoporosis if you have certain risk factors but don't have any apparent signs and symptoms. For example, you may be a middle-age woman with a family history of osteoporosis, but you haven't broken a bone, lost height or experienced any sudden-onset back pain. You should consider being screened for osteoporosis at least once during your lifetime. Be aware, though, that there is some controversy among doctors as to exactly when a screening test should be done.

Screening for low bone density is done with bone densitometry. You don't need a referral from your doctor. You can perform the test yourself with a small densitometer, which may be available at certain retail locations in your neighborhood. If the test results of your screening are normal, keep doing the right things to keep your bones healthy. If the test results suggest your bones are weaker than they should be for your age and sex, consider contacting your doctor for more in-depth testing.

Diagnostic tests

Diagnostic tests are performed on someone who is suspected of having a disorder because of the presence of signs and symptoms and certain risk factors. Diagnostic tests are often more precise, and more expensive, than screening tests. If you're 40 or older and you break a bone, you'll likely undergo diagnostic testing for osteoporosis. The primary diagnostic tools are the bone density test and a complete examination known as a history and physical evaluation.

You'll learn later in this chapter why a history and physical evaluation is so important for making a diagnosis.

Diagnostic tests are done to:

- Confirm that you have osteoporosis
- Determine the severity of your low bone density
- Establish your baseline bone density values

Testing is arranged by your doctor and done with a more accurate densitometer than the one you may have used for screening.

What is a bone density test?

A bone density test is about as close as your doctor may come to foretelling the future of your bone health. By looking at the test results, he or she can tell if you have osteoporosis and give you a strong indication of your susceptibility to fracture.

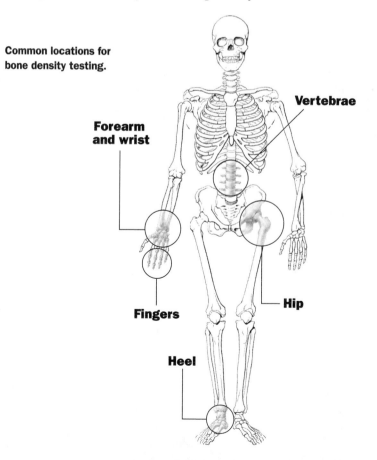

Common locations for bone density testing.

Vertebrae

Forearm and wrist

Fingers

Hip

Heel

A bone density test is simple, fast and painless. It uses special X-rays to measure how many grams of calcium and other bone minerals — collectively known as bone mineral content — are packed into a square centimeter of bone. A gram is about $\frac{1}{28}$ of an ounce. A centimeter is about a half inch. The terms *bone mineral content* and *bone density* are often used interchangeably. The higher your mineral content, the denser your bones. The denser your bones, the stronger they are and the less likely they are to break.

Bone density tests are usually done on bones that you're most likely to break because of osteoporosis. These sites include the lumbar vertebrae, which are in the lower region of your spine, the narrow neck of your femur bone adjoining the hip, and the bones of your wrist or forearm.

Who should be tested?

Ideally, adults considered at risk of osteoporosis will have their bone density tested. Early testing gives them more time to start preventive measures and allow the measures to work. It's also the first and best step toward receiving a diagnosis and being treated. Remember: If the development of osteoporosis can be slowed, then prevention is your goal.

It's recommended that the following individuals have a bone density test:

- All adult women before age 65.
- Anyone over 40 who has broken a bone and is willing to undergo treatment for osteoporosis.
- All women, men and children who are at high risk of osteoporosis. Being at high risk is generally considered as having two or more risk factors.
- All women, men and children who are taking or will soon take corticosteroid drugs.
- All young adults who for any reason have a low estrogen or testosterone level.
- All adults who have a medical condition known to lower bone mass and increase the risk of fractures.

If you're a woman, consider being tested before you reach menopause, even if you have no risk factors. Menopause generally

---

What does bone density tell you?

A bone density test provides a snapshot of the mineral content of a section of a specific bone at a single moment in time. This snapshot can:

- Determine if you have low bone density at specific parts of your skeleton, whether or not you've broken a bone there
- Determine if you have osteoporosis

If you're tested at intervals of a year or more, the results can be compared and used to:

- Identify changes in bone density that may be occurring over time
- Determine how your bone density is responding to treatment

---

occurs around age 50. An earlier test is advisable if you're at high risk of osteoporosis or if you've broken a bone or are losing height.

Any postmenopausal woman who breaks a bone should be tested because osteoporosis will be a primary suspect for causing the fracture. If osteoporosis is the cause, the test can determine how severely you have the condition.

Bone density testing is usually not a one-time thing. Even if your bone density is normal at the initial test, plan to be retested in about 5 years. Bone density tests taken at intervals over several years can reveal the rate at which you may be losing bone. The rate of bone loss is a potent predictor of your fracture risk.

The frequency of retesting depends on your age and the factors that put you at risk. One to 2 years is the minimum amount of time for bone affected by osteoporosis to show a noticeable increase or decrease in density. If you're taking medicine to treat osteoporosis, you may benefit from an annual bone density test during the first couple of years of treatment until it's clear your bone mass is stable. Thereafter, the tests can be less frequent. If you're taking corticosteroids, it's recommended that you be tested once a year.

Only a small fraction of adults who have osteoporosis or are at risk of it are properly screened, diagnosed and treated. Part of the reason is that not enough people are getting bone density tests. In a

study of 34,000 women over age 50, only 2 percent of the participants had ever had a bone density test. This was in spite of the fact
that 44 percent of the women had one or more risk factors for low
bone density.

How do you get tested?

Perhaps the best way to arrange a bone density test is through your
personal physician. He or she may not always consider giving you
a bone density test during a regular physical exam or office visit, so
it may be up to you to call it to your doctor's attention. Don't be
shy about inquiring about a test, particularly if you've broken a
bone, are nearing menopause or simply want to be screened.

Most tests take place in hospitals, usually in the radiology
department. Some hospitals have special osteoporosis programs,
often as part of a women's health center. Some larger cities have
osteoporosis centers unaffiliated with a hospital. If you don't have a
personal physician, any hospital in your community can help you
find one. Endocrinologists — doctors who specialize in the body's
hormonal system — also are specially trained to screen, diagnose
and treat osteoporosis. Someone with this background would be a
good choice to consider.

But you don't need a doctor's order to get the test. You can get
one on your own, using a peripheral bone densitometer. However,
this is less accurate than the devices often used at hospitals. The
peripheral devices are becoming widely available at drugstores,
malls, health fairs and other convenient locations. These devices
won't determine if you have osteoporosis, but they do provide
enough information for screening and an indication of whether
additional testing is needed.

How do you pay for testing?

Bone density tests can cost from $5 to $200, depending on where
you get tested and what type of device is used. Some health insurance plans pay for the tests, and others don't. You may need to ask
your health plan administrator if bone density testing is covered
and, if so, how much of the cost is paid. This information may also
be available in your benefit summary booklet.

Private insurance plans often follow Medicare guidelines for how much they pay. Coverage may also depend on whether the procedure is labeled a screening test or a diagnostic test. Your test is often considered a screening if you have no signs or symptoms and the results show you don't have osteoporosis. If you have signs or symptoms, the test is usually considered diagnostic.

Government assistance for bone density testing

Both Medicare and Medicaid pay for bone density tests under specific circumstances. How much they pay varies greatly, depending on where you live.

Medicare. Medicare is the federal health insurance program for individuals age 65 and older who receive Social Security benefits. At the present time, the program pays for bone density tests for:

- Women age 65 and older, especially those not taking medications to prevent bone loss
- Women and men whose X-rays show a previous spine fracture
- Women and men currently taking or planning to go on corticosteroids
- Women and men who have been diagnosed with primary hyperparathyroidism
- Women and men monitoring their condition to see if osteoporosis treatment is working

For more information, visit the official Medicare Web site: *www.medicare.gov.*

Medicaid. Medicaid is a federal program that helps pay medical costs for low-income Americans and people with certain disabilities. It's known in some states as medical assistance. This program is administered by each state's individual welfare system, so the benefits and eligibility requirements vary from state to state. For more information, contact the accounts payable department at your local clinic or a social service agency within your state government. Also visit the Centers for Medicare & Medicaid Services Web site: *www.cms.gov.*

How do bone densitometers work?

Bone density testing uses a device called a bone densitometer. Most densitometers measure the absorption of a low-energy X-ray beam as it passes through bone. The amount of X-ray energy (photons) that enters the bone is compared with the amount of energy that leaves the bone. And the denser the bone, the more of the X-ray beam that's absorbed.

Why not use regular X-rays for a bone density test? Regular X-rays are higher energy and optimal for a wide variety of imaging. But the energy of regular X-rays isn't sensitive enough to detect low bone density until a bone has lost 25 percent to 40 percent of its mineral content. By then you may already have osteoporosis in an advanced stage.

Radiation exposure from X-ray beams used for bone density testing is very low — only a fraction of the radiation used for a standard chest X-ray. You usually don't have to wear a protective apron, and the person testing you doesn't need to leave the room.

All bone density tests are quick, painless and noninvasive, which means nothing is put inside your body during the testing. Usually, tests take 1 to 15 minutes, depending on the type of densitometer being used. This doesn't include the time needed for filling out forms and other prep work.

At the hospital a radiologist, endocrinologist or other bone specialist will assess your test results. In most cases, you'll hear the results directly from your regular doctor. If they show bone loss, he or she can prescribe a treatment plan to slow bone loss if it's caused by aging or menopause. If overactive parathyroid glands or another secondary cause is responsible for your bone loss, your doctor may refer you to an endocrinologist.

Types of bone densitometers

Several types of bone densitometers of varying sizes and levels of accuracy are available. Some work best to measure the bone density of specific bones.

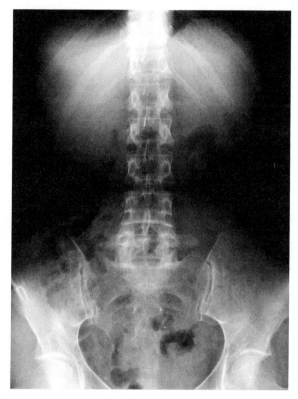

Bones of different densities will appear differently on an X-ray image. This image of the pelvis and spine shows areas of denser bone (lighter areas) and more porous bone (darker areas).

Central densitometers

Central densitometers are relatively large — large enough for you to lie down on — and usually are found in hospitals or the offices of bone disease specialists. As the name might suggest, these instruments are often used to measure the density of the central, stabilizing parts of your skeleton, such as the spine and hip. But they can also be used on any bone in the body. Central densitometers provide the most accurate bone density tests and are good predictors of your potential risk of fracture. The tests usually cost from $125 to $200. Two types of central densitometry are dual energy X-ray absorptiometry and quantitative computerized tomography:

Dual energy X-ray absorptiometry (DEXA). This procedure is the most accurate way to measure your bone density, so doctors usually rely on DEXA to diagnose osteoporosis. The use of two dif-

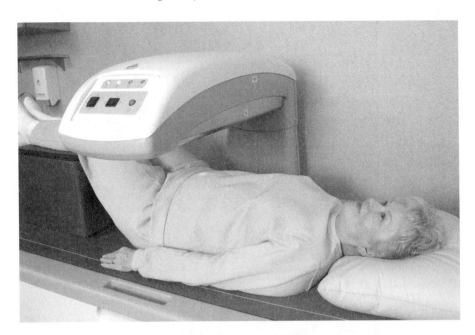

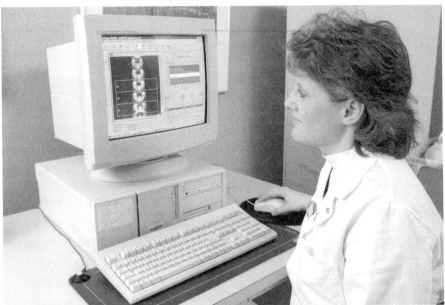

Dual energy X-ray absorptiometry (DEXA) is the most accurate procedure to screen or diagnose for osteoporosis. To measure the density of your spine, you'll lie flat on your back with your legs raised on a foam cube (above). The arm of the DEXA device positioned over your spine will detect energy from an X-ray source located under the table. This information is transmitted to a computer (below). An image of the bone will appear on the computer screen along with a summary table of bone density measurements and a graph that compares your measurements to a normal range for your age. For more information on bone density test results, see Chapter 6.

Bone scans and bone biopsies

Bone density tests aren't the same as bone scans or bone biopsies. Bone scans often are used to diagnose cancer or occasionally some rare bone diseases. A small amount of radioactive dye injected into your bloodstream collects in your bones, which allows a radiologist to see problem hot spots. Much as with a bone density test, your body's exposure to radiation from a bone scan is very small.

A bone biopsy is a procedure that uses a hollow needle to remove a small sample of bone tissue from your hip. This sample is tested to see if you have other bone diseases, such as osteomalacia (os-te-o-muh-LAY-shuh), which is a softening of the bones caused by a variety of other conditions.

---

ferent X-ray beams increases the precision of the measurement. This instrument can detect as little as a 3 percent to 5 percent change in bone density between successive scans. As you lie on a padded platform, mechanical arms that contain an X-ray source (under the table) and an X-ray detector (above your body) are properly aligned. The healthier your bone is, the less X-ray energy passes through it. The amount of X-ray energy absorbed by the bone is measured to determine your bone density. With the latest equipment, a DEXA test takes 3 to 6 minutes to obtain an accurate result.

DEXA is usually done on the lumbar vertebrae, which is the lower portion of your spine, and on the narrow neck of your femur bone, just below the hip joint. This part of your femur is the best predictor of a hip fracture, which is the most serious complication of osteoporosis. A DEXA test of the hip is often used to predict future fracture risk of other bones as well. Because of its accuracy, DEXA is the preferred test for a baseline bone density measurement for anyone starting medication to treat osteoporosis.

Quantitative computerized tomography (QCT). This procedure measures your bone density using computerized tomography. You lie on a movable padded table that slides into a large ring where the measurements are made. X-ray images are obtained from all angles. Special bone density computer software processes these images and combines them into a single scan that's useful for assessing bone structure. The test usually takes no more than 10 minutes.

QCT is most often used to measure density in your vertebrae and the portion of the femur bone below your hip. Test results are often used to monitor how well you're responding to treatment. A QCT test is more expensive than other densitometers and exposes you to more radiation.

Peripheral densitometers

Peripheral densitometers are smaller and less expensive than central densitometers. They're used to measure bone density on the periphery of your skeleton, such as in your finger, wrist and heel bones. Peripheral densitometers aren't as accurate as the central devices in predicting your risk of hip fracture, but they're accurate enough to screen anyone at risk of osteoporosis.

You can find peripheral devices in some drugstores and other retail locations, set up for do-it-yourself use. Peripheral densitometry usually costs $20 to $40. Sometimes, this type of test is offered free or for only a few dollars as part of health fairs or store promotions. If the results of a peripheral test show that you have low bone density, you'll need to follow that up with a central densitometer test. This can provide a more accurate result and help you and your doctor determine what measures are necessary to either prevent or treat the condition. Several types of peripheral densitometry tests are available:

Quantitative ultrasound (QUS). This procedure is often called heel ultrasound because most often it measures the heel bone. Instead of X-ray radiation, QUS sends high-frequency sound waves through your heel while you rest your bare foot on the instrument. And rather than measure absorption, this type of densitometer measures the reflection of sound waves. The denser your bone, the sooner sound waves are reflected back to the device.

This is a newer type of densitometer — it's portable, low cost and widely available. It measures your bone density in less than 1 minute. QUS is an easy way to be screened if you think you're at risk of osteoporosis. It's not accurate enough to positively diagnose

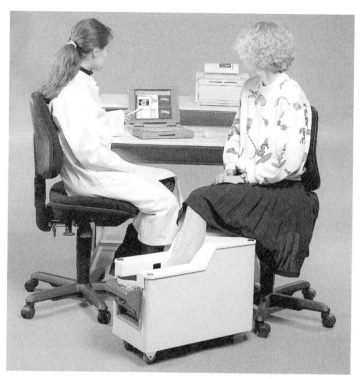

Quantitative ultrasound offers a fast, simple and accurate way to screen for osteoporosis.

osteoporosis or osteopenia of the central skeleton, or to assess the results of treatment.

Heel ultrasound is almost as accurate as DEXA at predicting your risk of breaking a hip or any other bone that's not part of the spine. But QUS can't measure changes in your central skeleton over time or tell if your bones are responding to medication. Because the heel bone is subjected to constant pressure from bearing the weight of your upper body, it's not a sensitive enough predictor of these types of bone mineral changes.

Peripheral dual energy X-ray absorptiometry (pDEXA). This procedure uses a compact, portable DEXA scanner. With the use of X-rays, pDEXA measures bone density in your finger, wrist or heel. This test takes about 3 minutes and is accurate enough to screen anyone at risk of osteoporosis.

Peripheral quantitative computerized tomography (pQCT). This rarely used procedure utilizes a small, portable QCT machine to measure the bone density of your wrist or hand. While seated

Types of bone densitometers

Technique	Abbreviation	Common testing location
Central		
Dual energy X-ray absorptiometry	DEXA	Spine, hip, forearm and total body
Quantitative computerized tomography	QCT	Spine and hip
Peripheral		
Quantitative ultrasound	QUS	Heel
Peripheral dual energy X-ray absorptiometry	pDEXA	Finger, wrist or heel
Peripheral quantitative computerized tomography	pQCT	Wrist or forearm
Radiographic absorptiometry	RA	Wrist or hand

with your hand, wrist or forearm placed inside the machine, X-rays pass through your bone, and the pQCT calculates your bone density. The procedure takes about 10 minutes. These machines are used more widely in Europe than in the United States.

Radiographic absorptiometry (RA). This procedure uses ordinary X-rays to measure bone density in your wrist or hand. Because ordinary X-rays aren't as sensitive as those used by other types of densitometers, a small aluminum plate — called a step wedge — is placed next to your hand as a bone density reference. Test results compare the density of your bone with the density of the aluminum. The procedure takes 2 or 3 minutes.

Which test is right for you?

Which type of bone density test is best for you depends on your age and on why you're being tested. Perhaps you're concerned because you have risk factors that make you susceptible to osteoporosis. Maybe you're worried about how strong a particular bone is. Or maybe you have no risk factors but are simply curious. Here's a guide that can help you with your decision:

If you have no risk factors. If you have no risk factors for osteoporosis and haven't broken a bone, a less expensive peripheral screening test, such as a pDEXA or QUS, is generally sufficient. If the results show low bone density, you and your doctor will likely follow up with tests from a more accurate central densitometer, such as a DEXA.

If you're worried about the strength of a specific bone, be tested with the device that most accurately measures that part of your skeleton. Your doctor can advise you. If you're concerned about the overall risk of fracture anywhere in your body, the best predictor is a DEXA of the femur neck that adjoins your hip.

If you have multiple risk factors or have broken a bone. If you suspect that you may have osteoporosis, your doctor can arrange for a DEXA test — even if the result of an earlier peripheral test was normal. A woman younger than age 65 is more likely to suffer a vertebral fracture, so a DEXA of the spine may be the most accurate indicator. In women age 65 or older, hip fractures are increasingly common, so a DEXA of the hip may reveal more.

DEXA can measure bone density accurately in other parts of your skeleton. That's good because osteoporosis tends to affect different parts of your skeleton at different times. In addition, different parts of a skeleton lose bone at different rates, particularly in postmenopausal women. For these reasons, it's often a good idea to test more than one location. Your bone density may be normal at one site but low at another.

If secondary osteoporosis is suspected. Secondary osteoporosis can be attributed to a known cause, such as a disease, a surgical procedure or a medication. Your doctor will select a testing procedure based on what he or she thinks may be causing the bone loss. If, for example, you have hyperparathyroidism, you may be losing mostly cortical bone, in which case a DEXA of your forearm may be the best choice because your forearm is made mostly of cortical bone.

If you've received a diagnosis of osteoporosis. If you have osteoporosis, your doctor may schedule periodic DEXA tests of your hip, spine and wrist, which are the primary fracture sites. When testing is done over several years, the best results come from the same densitometer operated by the same technician testing the same bone. That's because test results are slightly different for each machine. Densitometry experts are still trying to come up with a way to compare test results from different densitometers.

If you're monitoring the effects of medication. If you're taking medication such as bisphosphorates or teraperatide, central densitometry of your spine is best. The trabecular bone in your spine best shows the effects of medication. Peripheral densitometry would be of little use because it's not accurate enough to provide this information.

History and physical evaluation

Many people mistakenly believe that a bone density test is all you need to diagnose osteoporosis. It's true that the test can confirm you have low bone density, but can it tell you why? Is there anything about your general health or lifestyle that's making matters worse? To answer this question, you'll need a complete medical evaluation including a history and physical.

A history and physical is a thorough examination of your body systems and organs. You'll also likely have some blood and urine tests. Be prepared to describe any health concerns if you have them. During the exam, your doctor will ask you questions about your personal medical history and the medical history of your close relatives. You'll be asked about medications you're taking, what you eat, how much you exercise, and how much tobacco and alcohol you use. Be honest with your answers. Your doctor isn't there to judge you but to determine your risk of osteoporosis and to identify other conditions that may cause the symptoms.

What will your doctor know at the end of a history and physical evaluation? For starters, he or she will have identified or eliminated any number of conditions that could be secondary causes of osteoporosis. The evaluation also helps your doctor decide if you need another bone density test, which parts of your skeleton should be tested and which type of densitometer should be used. A history and physical evaluation also helps your doctor interpret the results of your bone density test. Without a history and physical, your test may not be as useful or may even be misinterpreted.

Bone marker tests

Bone marker tests measure bone turnover, that is, the rate at which bone changes. Test results don't indicate in which direction the remodeling cycle is headed — whether you're losing more bone or growing more bone — only that there's change. These results aren't always the type of information that your doctor will need to understand your bone health. So marker tests are used less often than bone density tests in diagnosing and treating osteoporosis.

Here's how a bone marker test works. The bone-remodeling cycle releases chemical byproducts into your bloodstream and urine. These byproducts are remnants of the material that make up your bone as well as hormones and enzymes associated with the remodeling cycle. Test results indicate the rate at which bone breakdown (resorption) and formation are occurring. If it's known that you're losing bone at the time a bone marker test is given, a high rate of bone turnover means faster bone loss.

Bone marker tests can't be used to diagnose osteoporosis, and they aren't used in the day-to-day management of this condition. These tests are not a substitute for bone density tests.

Who should have a bone marker test?

What you read about bone marker tests may make them sound like routine procedures — that you can walk into your doctor's office and ask for one. That's not the case. The fact is you probably don't need a marker test if you have the most common types of osteoporosis, which are associated with aging and menopause. Your doctor may recommend a bone marker test only if he or she wants to determine if you have an accelerated rate of bone turnover.

Bone marker tests are most useful if your bone loss is associated with a medical condition whose effect on your skeleton is not known. Bone markers may indicate if that condition is affecting bone turnover. These tests can also be useful for monitoring your treatment for that condition.

Bone marker tests usually aren't good at predicting fracture risk, although sometimes they can be used when the results are compared with a bone density test of the hip. Postmenopausal women who have the highest rates of bone turnover tend to have the highest rates of bone loss.

Types

Some bone marker tests measure byproducts of bone formation, and others measure byproducts of bone breakdown. Some measure byproducts in your urine, and others measure them in your blood. Marker tests are minimally painless and noninvasive. But many factors — including your diet, the time of day that the test is administered and, in women, the menstrual cycle — influence these tests and limit their usefulness.

Making a diagnosis

Of the tools your doctor has for diagnosing osteoporosis, the bone density test combined with a history and physical is the most important. A DEXA scan of the hip is usually the best bone density test to calculate your fracture risk and, based on this information, determine if you have osteoporosis. The history and physical determines your general state of health and may help your doctor detect a possible disorder that could cause osteoporosis. Bone marker tests also may alert your doctor to a secondary cause.

After your bone density test, you'll probably have a follow-up visit with your doctor to discuss the test results. You'll get more out of that discussion if you understand what all of the numbers and lines on your printout mean. You can learn more about this in the next chapter.

Chapter 6

Making sense of your test results

Let's say you've had a bone density test. You get the results and — good grief — look at all of the numbers and lines! What do they mean? Although bone density is not the only factor that determines bone strength, it's the only factor that can be measured. Those seemingly incomprehensible numbers and lines on your printout can give your doctor an accurate measure of your bone density and insight into the health of your skeleton.

That's why bone density tests are so important to doctors in determining whether or not to make a diagnosis of osteoporosis. Remember that a bone density test measures how much mineral content, such as calcium and phosphate, is packed into a square centimeter of bone. The denser your bones, the stronger your bones and the less likely they are to break. Well-defined criteria have been developed for interpreting the measurements. Two numbers from the test results that draw the most attention are your T-score and your Z-score.

A bone density test can also be a good predictor of your risk of breaking a bone. Very low bone density at any site on your skeleton means the chances of breaking a bone there or somewhere else is high. For example, if a bone density test of your hip is low, the chance of breaking your hip is high, and the chance of fracturing a vertebra is also high.

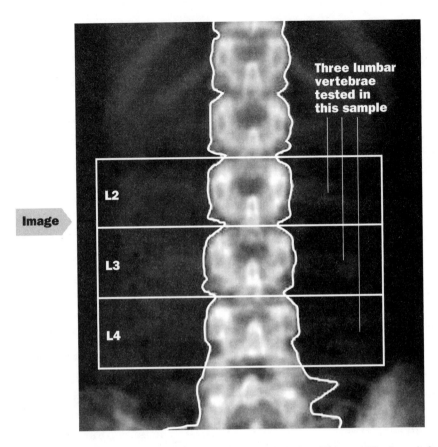

Main elements from a bone density test of the spine include an image of the bone being tested (above) and a summary table and graph (adjoining page). This DEXA test indicates someone in his or her early 40s with good bone density of the lumbar region of the spine.

What you see on your test results

Your bone density test results will include at least three elements: a black-and-white image, a summary table of bone density numbers, and a graph. These elements are what a physician sees on the computer screen while performing your bone density test.

The black-and-white image is a graphic representation of bone density. The example above shows that this test was performed on the spine. White rectangles are superimposed over the image of three of the vertebrae. The labels L2, L3 and L4 indicate that, for this test, bone density was measured on the second, third and fourth vertebrae in the lumbar region of the spine.

	Region	Bone density	Young-adult T-score	Age-matched Z-score
Summary table	L2	1.270	0.6	1.1
	L3	1.243	0.4	0.9
	L4	1.301	0.8	1.3
	L2-L4	1.272	0.6	1.1

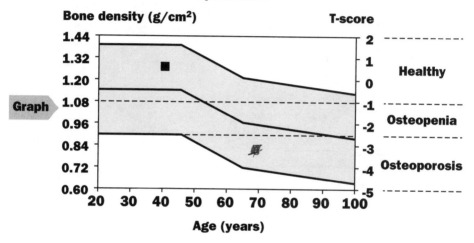

Spine L2-L4

Graph

Normal range of bone density for lumbar vertebrae over time.

The L2, L3 and L4 labels also appear in the summary table from this example. The second column is where you'll find the actual bone density values for each vertebra that has been measured. Other columns indicate what are known as T-scores and Z-scores. Their meanings are explained later in the chapter. The numbers on the bottom row are an average for the three vertebrae combined.

The graph compares the average bone density for the three lumbar vertebrae (L2 to L4) with a normal range for your age. The shaded area crossing the graph portrays this normal range. The position of the black square on the graph indicates that the person being tested is in his or her early 40s with a bone density of around 1.27 (the table shows the value is exactly 1.272). This person has

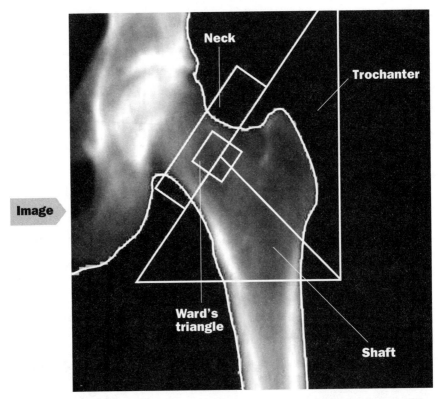

A DEXA test of the hip will have the same three elements as a bone density test of the spine: an image, summary table and graph. The four regions of the hip measured in this test are indicated on the image (above) by white outlines. The names for the Ward's triangle and trochanter regions are abbreviated on the summary table (right) as *Wards* and *Troch* respectively. Test results indicate someone in his or her early 40s with good bone density of the left femur.

excellent bone density in the lumbar region, with a score in the upper half of the range for individuals around age 40.

Bone density test results from other locations on your skeleton will include elements similar to the test results of the spine. The example above shows a bone density test result for the left hip. The black square on the graph indicates a 40-year-old person with normal bone density of the hip for his or her age. White lines superimposed on the image indicate four different regions of the femur where bone density is measured. They are called the neck, shaft, trochanter (tro-KAN-tur) and Ward's triangle (which is actually square on the image). The summary table lists each region individually and provides an average score of the four regions (total).

Region	Bone density	Young-adult T-score	Age-matched Z-score
Neck	0.919	-0.5	0.0
Wards	0.734	-1.4	-0.8
Troch	0.724	-0.6	-0.2
Shaft	1.118	-	-
Total	0.932	-0.6	-0.1

Summary table

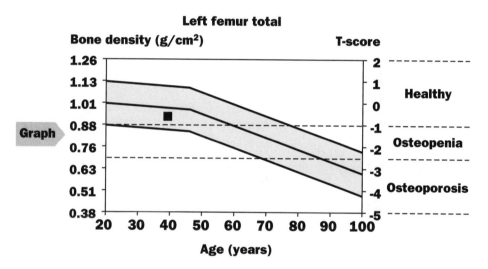

Left femur total

Normal range of bone density for the left femur over time.

How do these tests results indicate if someone has osteoporosis? Look at the example on page 76 of the graph from a bone density test of the spine. The black square on the graph indicates a person around 80 years of age. His or her bone density score for the lumbar region of the spine is around 0.75. This person is in the low range for his or her age and would be diagnosed with osteoporosis.

What hasn't been explained from these examples are T-scores and Z-scores. Both scores provide important information to your doctor. And the T-score figures prominently in any diagnosis of osteoporosis. There's variation in how these numbers are derived among different densitometers. The sections that follow will help you understand what the scores mean and how they're used.

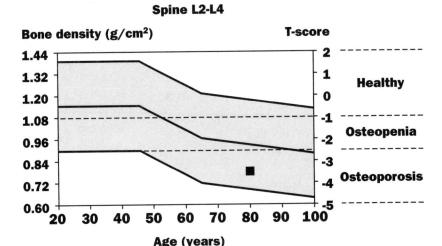

Spine L2-L4

This graph from a bone density test of the spine indicates someone around 80 years old who would be diagnosed as having osteoporosis.

Understanding T-scores

If you're a woman, your T-score compares your bone density with that of a large group of young women of your weight and race at peak bone mass who have normal, healthy bone density. If you're a man, your T-score compares your bone density with that of young men of your weight and race who have normal, healthy bone density.

You might be wondering why a bone density test compares you with a group of women or men who may be considerably younger than you. Many people with osteoporosis are 60 or older. This type of comparison may not seem fair or even useful, but there's actually a good reason for doing it this way. It allows for everybody to be compared with a common baseline — a normal, young population at the age of peak bone mass, which is usually between the ages of 30 and 40. No one expects a 60-year-old woman to have the same T-score as someone at peak bone mass. Value comes from comparing everyone with the same standard.

The actual number on your test result represents the difference between your bone density and the average bone density, or mean value, of young, healthy adults of your sex. The number expresses

Region	Bone density	Young-adult T-score	Age-matched Z-score
L2	1.270	0.6	1.1
L3	1.243	0.4	0.9
L4	1.301	0.8	1.3
L2-L4	1.272	0.6	1.1

T-score referred to for diagnosis

The third and fourth columns on this table indicate the T-scores and Z-scores for the three vertebrae measured in this test. The bottom T-score — the average score of all three vertebrae — is the one a doctor would consider most heavily for a diagnosis of osteoporosis. A T-score of +0.6 is higher than average by more than one-half of a standard deviation.

how much you differ (deviate) from this mean value. If your T-score is 0.0, you don't deviate at all from the norm because you match the group you're being compared with. If your T-score is -1.0, your bone density is lower than average by one standard deviation. Likewise, if your T-score is +0.5, your bone density is higher than average by one-half of a standard deviation.

To determine whether to give you a diagnosis of osteopenia or osteoporosis based strictly on bone density testing, your doctor will interpret your T-score following the official guidelines of the World Health Organization (WHO) and the National Osteoporosis Foundation (NOF):

- If your T-score is within one standard deviation of the average, that is, between +1.0 and -1.0, you have normal bone density.
- If your T-score is -1.0 to -2.5 standard deviations below the average, you have low bone density, a condition known as osteopenia.
- If your T-score is at least -2.5 or lower than the average, you have osteoporosis.
- If your T-score is at least -2.5 or lower than the average and you have broken one or more bones, you have severe osteoporosis.

The same criteria apply to men and women. For most bone density tests, a -1.0 standard deviation equals a 10 percent to 12 percent decrease in bone density. So a T-score of -2.5 would mean your bone density is about 25 percent to 30 percent lower than that of average healthy women or men at their peak bone mass.

T-scores from different bones in your skeleton can't be compared. Generally, when more than one bone is tested, doctors use the lowest T-score to diagnose osteoporosis. For example, if you have a T-score of -2.7 in your spine and a T-score of -2.0 in your hip, the spine T-score would be used to indicate that you have osteoporosis.

Test results may be a good indicator of osteoporosis, but they're not a complete diagnosis. Being told that you have osteopenia (a T-score in the range of -1.0 to -2.5) doesn't guarantee that you'll eventually develop osteoporosis but it does mean that a further decline in your bone density must be avoided. That's why your doctor's input is so important.

Understanding Z-scores

Your Z-score compares your bone density with that of an average group of women or men who are approximately your age and of similar weight and same race who have not been diagnosed with osteoporosis. Although your Z-score is a good indicator of how normal or abnormal your bone density is for your age, it's not used to determine if you have osteoporosis. A T-score is used for that. Your doctor will refer to criteria for the T-score established by the World Health Organization to make a diagnosis.

Your Z-score is useful because it may suggest you have a secondary form of osteoporosis — whether something other than aging or menopause is causing abnormal bone loss. A Z-score lower than -1.5 means secondary osteoporosis may be suspect. Your physician will then try to determine if there's an underlying cause for the low bone mass. If a cause can be identified, that condition can often be treated and the bone loss slowed or stopped.

In general, the lower your Z-score, the more likely something other than aging or menopause is contributing to bone loss. But fewer than 3 percent of adults have a Z-score lower than -2.0. Fewer than 1 percent have a Z-score lower than -3.0.

You may have a normal Z-score and an abnormal T-score. This is quite common among older adults. That's because everyone loses bone density as they age. By the time many people reach their 80s, their bone density will be normal for their age according to the Z-score, but they may have osteopenia or osteoporosis, according to the T-score.

How are the numbers used?

The T-scores and Z-scores are important pieces of information from your bone density test results. Now that you have a basic understanding of how the scores are calculated, let's look at two imaginary examples that illustrate how the numbers are used to assess bone health and diagnose osteoporosis.

Example 1

Ms. J is 59 years old. She has completed menopause. She doesn't smoke and doesn't drink alcohol in excess. She doesn't take corticosteroids and has never broken a bone. Her mother had osteoporosis. Concerned about her own chances of getting the disease,

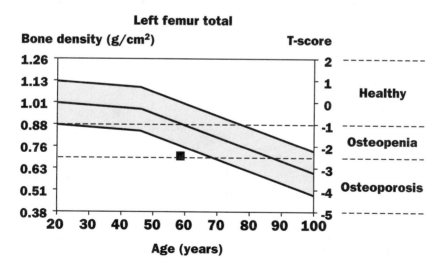

Ms. J's bone density test of the hip.

Ms. J talks to her doctor. Given her age and family history, her doctor arranges for Ms. J to have a bone density test of her hip using dual energy X-ray absorptiometry (DEXA).

Ms. J studies a graph on the printout of her test results. She notices how normal bone density for the left femur gradually declines and becomes more pronounced at about age 40. A black square on the graph shows that her T-score is -2.3. That means her bone density is 2.3 standard deviations below the mean value of a group of healthy, young women with approximately her weight and of the same race. Although she doesn't have osteoporosis — which would be indicated with a T-score of -2.5 or lower — she is told she has osteopenia and is at risk of osteoporosis if she experiences bone loss in the future.

Ms. J's Z-score is -0.7, which means her bone density is less than the norm for women her age by seven-tenths of a standard deviation. Her Z-score is not low enough to suggest she has a secondary cause for her bone loss.

Example 2

Ms. K is 42 year old. Seven years ago, she had a total hysterectomy, which is the surgical removal of the uterus and ovaries. She wasn't given estrogen after surgery. She doesn't smoke or drink alcohol in

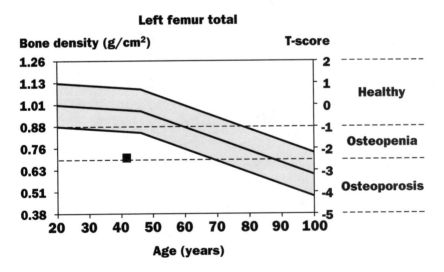

Ms. K's bone density test of the hip.

excess. She has no family history of osteoporosis and has never broken a bone. Ms. K's T-score is -2.3, the same as Ms. J's. But Ms. K is 15 years younger, which gives her an additional 15 years to lose more bone mass. For this reason, she is at greater risk of developing osteoporosis.

Ms. K's Z-score is -2.3, the same as her T-score. Such a low Z-score suggests something besides natural aging or menopause is affecting her bone density. In Ms. K's case, surgical menopause caused by her hysterectomy, and the attendant drop in estrogen level, may have triggered a sudden and early loss of bone density.

These two examples illustrate how similar bone density scores can have a different meaning for different people. You may have the same T-score as your neighbor, but one of you may develop osteoporosis and the other may not. Although Ms. K doesn't have osteoporosis, she's at much greater risk of getting it than Ms. J is because she's younger and has more time to lose bone.

Can test results predict a fracture?

In general, the lower your T-score, the higher your risk of fracture. As a rule of thumb, for every standard deviation below the normal peak bone mass, your risk of fracture approximately doubles. For example, if your T-score is -2.0, you're four times as likely to break a bone. Among men and women who have the same bone density, this risk of fracture is the same. A T-score of -2.5 — considered the boundary between osteopenia and osteoporosis — is defined by the WHO as the point below which treatment is necessary. But in fact, the -2.5 score is not an absolute boundary.

Though it's true that nothing can foretell the future with certainty, the T-score reveals more about fracture risk than a blood pressure reading tells of stroke risk or a cholesterol score reveals about heart attack risk. Still, keep in mind that having osteoporosis doesn't mean you'll definitely break a bone. It's like setting 140/90 millimeters of mercury (mm Hg) as the cutoff between high blood pressure and normal blood pressure. Just because your blood pressure is above that number doesn't mean you'll have a stroke. And there's no T-score below which you will definitely break a bone.

Z-scores also can help predict your risk of fracture. In general, if your Z-score is one standard deviation below the average for your age, your fracture risk doubles. It quadruples if it's two standard deviations below the average for your age. If you're an older adult and your Z-score is normal, you may still have low bone density and be at high risk of breaking a bone. Remember that normal for an older adult tends to be low when compared with a normal young adult.

Putting T-scores and Z-scores in context

T-scores and Z-scores are both statistical probabilities based on groups of people similar to you. But you're a unique individual with a specific genetic makeup and lifestyle that affect your risk. That's why your doctor considers other factors, including:

- Age
- Overall physical and emotional health
- Whether you've broken a bone in the past
- Medications you're taking or have taken in the past
- Family history
- Overall bone health

Your chance of breaking a bone naturally increases as you age, even if your bone density is normal. From age and daily wear and tear, your bones become more fragile and less able to absorb shock. If you've already broken a bone, you're at increased risk of breaking another bone. Studies indicate that 45 percent of 50-year-old women will fracture a hip, vertebra, forearm, wrist or other bone at some point in the remaining years of their lives. Many of these women won't have osteoporosis when they break the bone. For men in particular, the chances of breaking a bone increase greatly beyond age 75, no matter what their bone density is.

A bone density test doesn't measure bone quality. Bone quality is how connected and intact the structure of your bones is, not just the amount of material. Bone quality is another factor in how strong your bones are and how resistant they are to breaking. That means your bones may have low density but at the same time be of a high quality that resists breaking.

Important considerations

Some people make the mistake of thinking their T-score is all they need to know about their bone health. One number doesn't give the total picture. A T-score by itself can be easy to misinterpret or ignore. For example, you may have a normal T-score on your test results, but if you have a low-trauma compression fracture in your spine, you will still need to be concerned about osteoporosis. Other risk factors may be involved that would make your doctor decide to treat you for bone loss. The National Osteoporosis Foundation recommends that women with no risk factors other than their sex and age should be treated for osteoporosis if their T-score is -2.0 or lower.

Some people may have low T-scores but never fracture. For example, you may be a 60-year-old woman with a -3.0 T-score, which shows you have osteoporosis. But maybe you're also an avid tennis player, have been on medication to prevent bone loss since menopause and have never broken a bone. Your bone quality happens to be excellent because of good genes, healthy living and healthy eating. You may continue to live an active life with no ill effects from osteoporosis.

The future may be different if you have that same -3.0 T-score, but you're a 45-year-old woman, especially if you smoke, don't exercise and have already broken a bone. These circumstances put you at much higher risk of breaking a bone. And your doctor would treat your condition very differently.

The point is, T-scores and bone density tests in general aren't the be-all and end-all to understanding how lower bone mass affects you. There's more to your condition than a number from the densitometer. Before jumping to conclusions, always discuss your bone density test results with a doctor. It's important that your doctor connect all of the dots to give a complete picture of your bone health. He or she needs to assess your T-score in light of the other factors in your life that can affect your skeleton. Together you can decide how to treat bone loss with a strategy designed specifically for you. Learn more about what that strategy might involve in the next chapter.

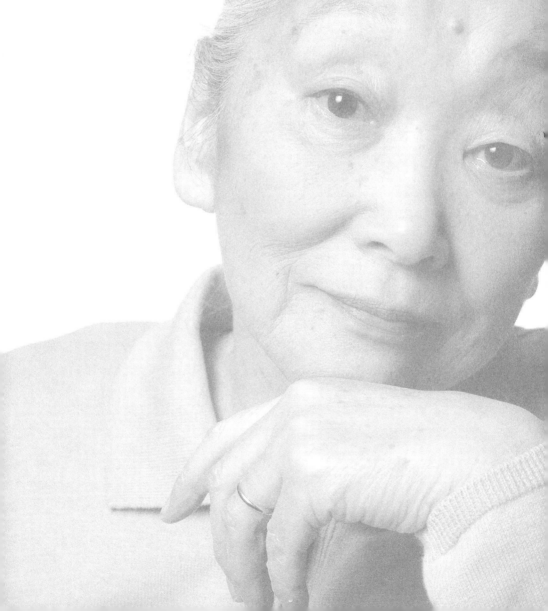

Part 2

Preventing and treating osteoporosis

Chapter 7

Elements of your action plan

It's never too early to start the battle against osteoporosis or too late to stop the condition in its tracks. Whether you're trying to prevent osteoporosis or treat it, the goal is the same: maintaining your bone health to ensure a low risk of fracture. And no matter your reason for setting this goal, the measures you'll take to achieve it are always the same. Many of these measures require your active participation.

Understanding your role in the prevention or treatment of osteoporosis is vital for success. This knowledge helps you coordinate key strategies related to factors such as diet, exercise and medications into a practical and achievable action plan. This action plan will be a blueprint designed specifically by you and your doctor to keep your bones healthy.

If you don't have osteoporosis, a prevention plan can greatly reduce your risk of getting the disease. Ideally, prevention begins in childhood and continues throughout life. The more you build up your bones during your early years, the less likely you are to develop osteoporosis later. But this isn't the only time an action plan can be effective. Even if you're an adult at increased risk or have been diagnosed with the condition, you can slow or put a stop to bone loss with effective use of the various strategies that you and your doctor work out together.

Strong bones for a lifetime

A successful action plan to prevent or treat osteoporosis involves several elements that contribute to overall bone health. These elements include good nutrition — including an adequate intake of calcium and vitamin D — regular physical activity, healthy habits and behaviors, good posture and medications. When combined, these elements support and strengthen one another to help you prevent or manage osteoporosis, keep you healthy and maintain your overall quality of life. Each element will be described in this chapter to show why it's so essential to your action plan and how it interrelates to other elements. Chapters 8 to 13 are each devoted to a different element, providing more detail and demonstrating how the strategies related to it can be put to practical use.

In establishing an action plan, consider these objectives:

- Maximize the development of your skeleton. As a child or young adult, the focus is on attaining a high peak bone mass. As an older adult, the goal is to stabilize existing bone mass.
- Prevent fractures. Bones weakened by the depletion of calcium and other minerals are more likely to break.
- Relieve the symptoms of fractures, stooped posture and chronic pain, should they occur.
- Improve your balance and the ability to move and be active.

Success in meeting these objectives depends in part on your commitment to the action plan. It's up to you to stick with daily routines and be willing to adapt some of your behaviors.

At the same time, you don't have to do it alone. In managing any chronic disease, it's important to maintain good relationships with and draw support from professionals, as well as from family and friends. Several kinds of doctors can help you, including endocrinologists, rheumatologists, general practitioners, internists, gynecologists, rehabilitation specialists and orthopedists. Often your own doctor is the best person to work with because he or she knows your medical history and special needs. In dealing with specific aspects of your action plan, you may find it useful to also consult a dietitian, physical or occupational therapist, social worker or mental health professional.

Starting young

The secret to preventing osteoporosis is to make your skeleton as strong as it can be by doing everything you can to help it reach its maximum peak bone mass. (For more discussion of peak bone mass, see Chapter 2.) By eating right and staying physically active during the years when bone mass is increasing — from childhood to approximately age 30 — you can lessen the impact of bone loss that occurs naturally in your later years.

Parents and grandparents can help children develop habits that will benefit their bones for the rest of their lives. Start by making sure children get enough calcium. Young people often have diets deficient in calcium. Good overall nutrition also is important. Some young women diet excessively in a quest to be thin and deprive themselves of valuable nutrients. Low body weight puts bones at risk. Conversely, studies show that young women can increase their bone mass by increasing calcium intake in their diet.

Many children love soft drinks, which have no calcium content. Parents can do their kids a favor by skipping the soda and offering milk or calcium-fortified juice instead. Milk and fruit juice are among the top sources of vitamins, calcium and magnesium for children in the United States.

Parents and grandparents can also encourage physical activity as part of the family routine, whether it's an evening walk after dinner, swimming, bowling, a canoe trip, or a game of basketball or tennis. Regular physical activity is essential for building strong muscles and bones.

Diet and nutrition

Good bone health starts with good nutrition — a well-balanced diet that includes enough calcium, vitamin D and other nutrients that your body needs to perform its daily functions. Calcium and vitamin D are essential nutrients for maximizing and preserving bone mass. Studies show that getting adequate amounts of calcium and vitamin D reduces the rate of bone loss that occurs with age and can reduce the risk of hip and nonvertebral fractures in older adults. Protein and other nutrients, such as the minerals phosphorus, sodium and magnesium, also play important roles in keeping your bones strong.

Calcium: The foundation

Calcium is found in every one of the billions of cells in your body, although about 99 percent of it lies in your skeleton. Because calcium is a major component of bone, you need adequate amounts of the mineral throughout your life to achieve and maintain peak bone mass. Calcium is also needed for your heart, muscles and nerves to function properly and for your blood to clot normally. Indeed, an adequate supply of calcium must always be available in your bloodstream. The body has built-in safeguards to regulate the calcium level in your blood — allowing neither too little nor too much.

Each day, you lose some calcium from your body in urine, feces and, to a lesser extent, sweat. This continual loss of calcium means that your body requires constant replenishment. If you don't consume enough of the mineral in your diet, your parathyroid glands will release a hormone that stimulates the release of calcium into circulation from your bones. Your bones give up the calcium in order to keep the calcium level in your blood normal. If this action occurs repeatedly over a long period of time, your bone density will decrease.

Calcium requirements. Calcium is essential during childhood and adolescence, when the skeleton is growing rapidly. But contrary to common belief, the need for dietary calcium actually increases with age. With aging, your body becomes less efficient at absorbing calcium and vitamin D from the diet and retaining calcium in the kidneys. For women, the drop in estrogen levels at menopause further reduces calcium absorption. In addition, many older adults eat fewer dairy products and other calcium-containing foods. They're also more likely to have chronic medical problems and use medications that may impair calcium absorption. All of these changes put greater pressure on your body to maintain sufficient calcium levels in your bloodstream.

Recommended daily intake of dietary calcium

Age	Adequate intake (milligrams/day)	Upper limit (milligrams/day)
0-6 months	210	
7-12 months	270	
1-3 years	500	2,500
4-8 years	800	2,500
9-18 years	1,300	2,500
19-50 years	1,000	2,500
51 years +	1,200	2,500

There is consensus among many physicians that a goal of 1,500 mg of calcium a day is reasonable for postmenopausal women.

Source: National Academy of Sciences, 2002

Unfortunately, many people aren't getting the calcium they need to keep their bones strong. The typical American diet provides less than 600 milligrams (mg) a day of calcium — well below recommended adult levels. Among children and adolescents, it's estimated that about 25 percent of boys and 10 percent of girls meet the recommended intakes. Only about 50 percent to 60 percent of older adults are getting the amount of calcium they need. So there's much a person can do to improve skeletal health at any age.

Researchers cite several possible reasons for this widespread calcium deficiency. Foremost is the fact that people are eating fewer dairy products. Some people avoid milk because of intolerance to lactose (the sugar in milk), fears of weight gain, or other reasons. In addition, people aren't eating enough fruits and vegetables, and they're consuming large amounts of high-phosphate, calcium-free beverages such as sodas.

One way to increase the calcium in your diet is to know which foods are rich in calcium and include them in your meals. Another way is to take a calcium supplement. These topics, as well as an overview of good nutrition, are discussed in Chapter 8.

Calcium requirements during pregnancy and lactation

During pregnancy a mother's body needs extra calcium for the developing fetus. To get additional calcium, the mother's ability to absorb the mineral from the intestines is increased — a nifty trick of Mother Nature. During lactation the mother's kidneys conserve calcium, making more available for her and the baby.

Because of these changes in the body, the recommended calcium intake for women during pregnancy and lactation is the same as that for all women of the same age. Nevertheless, if you're pregnant, talk to your doctor about meeting calcium requirements.

Vitamin D: Unlocking the door for calcium

Your calcium intake is not the whole story for strong bones. Your body must maintain a balance between how much calcium is absorbed from the food you eat and how much calcium is eliminated from your body.

Calcium absorption takes place as your intestines extract the mineral from food and move it into your bloodstream. Calcium excretion occurs primarily through urine, feces and sweat. Poor absorption and increased excretion can upset the calcium balance and weaken bones.

Vitamin D plays an important role in maintaining this balance by increasing calcium absorption in the small intestines. Vitamin D is like the key that unlocks a door, allowing calcium to leave the intestines and enter the bloodstream. If you don't get enough vitamin D, the level of calcium circulating in your bloodstream drops. That's when the parathyroid hormone signals your bones to release more calcium into circulation. Over time, a vitamin D deficiency results in abnormal bone loss.

Sources of vitamin D. An adequate supply of vitamin D requires exposure to sunlight. Ultraviolet (UV) radiation from the sun stimulates your skin to synthesize vitamin D. As much as 90 percent of your vitamin D supply can come from sunlight.

How much vitamin D you convert depends on many factors, including the season, the latitude at which you live, the amount of

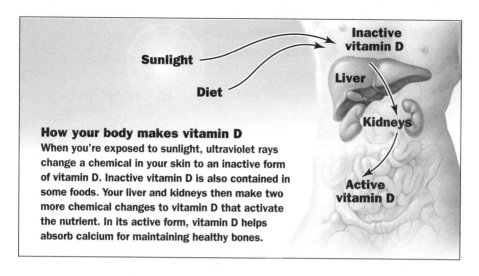

How your body makes vitamin D
When you're exposed to sunlight, ultraviolet rays change a chemical in your skin to an inactive form of vitamin D. Inactive vitamin D is also contained in some foods. Your liver and kidneys then make two more chemical changes to vitamin D that activate the nutrient. In its active form, vitamin D helps absorb calcium for maintaining healthy bones.

sunshine and air pollution in your region, your age, the condition of your skin, liver and kidneys, and the type of clothing you wear. Using sunscreen and spending long periods of time indoors prevent some people from getting the vitamin D they need. In northern latitudes, solar radiation isn't strong enough in the winter to produce adequate vitamin D in skin. During those months the body depends on its stored vitamin D or dietary sources.

Only a few foods are naturally rich in vitamin D. They include fatty fish, fish liver oils (including cod liver oil), liver and egg yolks. The milk you buy at the grocery store is usually fortified with vitamin D.

Vitamin D requirements. Getting enough vitamin D is necessary at any age. Most infants and children in the United States get enough vitamin D because it's added to milk. Although consumption of milk often decreases during adolescence, vitamin D deficiency is unusual in this age group.

Older adults are less likely to get enough vitamin D. With age, skin becomes less able to synthesize vitamin D, and organs such as the kidneys and liver may become less efficient at processing it. Older adults are less likely to consume foods fortified with vitamin D, such as milk. Their ability to absorb the vitamin from the food they eat also diminishes. Many older adults spend less time in the sun, particularly during the cold winter months in northern latitudes and with advancing age may become homebound.

Recommended daily intake of vitamin D

Age	Adequate intake (international units/day)	Upper limit (international units/day)
0-50 years	200	2,000
51-70 years	400-600	2,000
71 years +	600-800	2,000

Note: Amounts for vitamin D are sometimes expressed in micrograms (40 IU = 1 microgram).

Source: National Academy of Sciences, 2002

For adequate production of vitamin D from sunlight, some experts recommend getting 10 to 15 minutes of sun exposure on the face, arms and hands two to three times a week — depending on individual skin sensitivities. However, as mentioned above, many factors can reduce the effectiveness of sunlight for producing vitamin D. These include sunscreen, light filtered through a window, air pollution and the weakness of solar radiation in winter. If you're affected by any of these factors, you may benefit from vitamin D supplements. Individuals who take steroid medications such as prednisone or hydrocortisone may require additional vitamin D.

Other nutrients and your bones

Nutrients other than calcium and vitamin D may influence your bone health in both positive and negative ways.

Phosphorus. Phosphorus is present in most foods, including meat, poultry, fish, eggs, dairy products, nuts, legumes, cereals and grains. Phosphate salts are used extensively in processed foods. Phosphorus is important for the normal development and maintenance of your bones and tissues. But the intake of phosphorus in the American diet has risen 10 percent to 15 percent over the past 20 years, due primarily to the increased use of food additives and carbonated beverages. Unfortunately, an excess of phosphorus may have adverse effects on your skeleton.

Protein. Protein is one of the building blocks of bone and is essential for your body to build and repair tissue. It's also needed for fractures to heal and for the immune system to function properly. Most Americans consume more than the recommended amount of protein a day, which is 44 grams for women and 56 grams for men. For reference, 56 grams of protein is found in 2 cups of milk and 4 to 6 ounces of meat. Studies suggest that a high-protein diet may increase the amount of calcium excreted through your kidneys. On the other hand, a low-protein diet may interfere with calcium absorption in the intestines. A diet containing a moderate level of protein is probably best for you.

Sodium. Sodium chloride, the main component in table salt, increases calcium excretion through urine. Although unusual, a diet that is high in sodium may adversely affect the calcium balance in your bloodstream. Most American adults consume more than the recommended limit of 2,400 milligrams a day. Remember to taste your food before reaching for the salt shaker.

The bottom line? A well-balanced diet, including the recommended amounts of phosphorus, protein and sodium, is good for your bones. For more information about nutrition, see Chapter 8.

Body weight and osteoporosis

Most of us have heard about the dangers of being overweight, such as the increased risk of coronary artery disease and stroke. But being too lean also can be unhealthy, especially for your bones. It's important that your diet include enough calories to maintain a normal body weight because weight has a powerful impact on bone mass. Because weight increases the load on your skeleton, your bones compensate by growing stronger.

Women who are excessively lean run the risk of having low bone mass, excessive bone loss at menopause and a susceptibility to fracture. It's best to maintain a healthy, normal weight — neither overweight nor underweight. Adding weight beyond a normal range may suit your bones but increases many other health risks. If you're having trouble with your weight or your diet, talk to your doctor.

Physical activity

Being physically active on a regular basis is another key component of any action plan to prevent or treat osteoporosis. Studies show that plenty of physical activity early in life helps you achieve a higher peak bone mass. Regular exercise during your adult years can help slow bone loss, maintain your posture and strengthen your cardiovascular health. It also improves your balance, coordination and muscle strength, all of which reduce the risk of falling and breaking a bone. Evidence also indicates that physical activity improves muscle function. All of these factors help delay the loss of independence for many older adults, allowing them to maintain the lifestyle they want for a longer period of time and contributing to a higher quality of life.

Bone is living tissue that can strengthen — or weaken — in relation to how much it's used. The greater the demands you place on bone, the stronger and denser it becomes. When you perform an action such as hitting a tennis ball or landing on your feet after a jump, chemical messengers instruct your arm bones or leg bones to be ready to handle that impact again. Repeating the action over time reinforces the preparedness of your bones. If you look closely at X-rays of the arms of a tennis player, you can see that the bones of the dominant arm — the one that holds the racket — are larger and denser than the bones of the other arm. Conversely, people who are put on bed rest or otherwise immobilized lose bone strength quickly due to lack of activity and disuse.

Every bit of activity helps. Being active includes all the motions of going about your daily chores, running errands and simply living your life. It may also involve a more structured exercise program. You might choose to do weight-bearing exercises, such as walking, jogging, basketball and dancing, and resistance exercises, which often involve the use of weights. Other exercises are intended to strengthen your back muscles and improve your posture. Often a combination of these exercises is recommended for your action plan. Plan to talk with your doctor about what types of activities are appropriate for you. Physical activity is discussed in more detail in Chapter 9.

Medications

In addition to diet and exercise, medications are often prescribed for people at high risk of developing osteoporosis and those who have been diagnosed with the disease. As with the other components of an action plan, the main goal in using medications is to preserve or increase bone density and prevent fractures.

Most prescription medications for osteoporosis are called antiresorptives. The term refers to the action of slowing or stopping the breakdown of bone tissue (resorption). These medications don't affect bone formation — the other half of the bone-remodeling cycle. By putting the brakes on bone removal, antiresorptives help bone formation keep pace. This should slow bone loss and often allow bone density to increase over time.

A new drug recently tested and approved by the Food and Drug Administration functions in an opposite manner. Medication derived from parathyroid hormone works to build new bone and increase bone mass. It's called an anabolic agent. The word *anabolic* describes a process that promotes the formation of new tissue. The drug will be used to treat women and men with severe forms of osteoporosis, including those who are at a high risk of fracture and who haven't responded well to other forms of treatment, such as the antiresorptive drugs. For more detailed information about these medications, as well as medications under investigation, see Chapter 10.

Healthy behaviors

Along with a well-balanced diet, regular physical activity and medications, you may need to direct your attention to certain behaviors that you've practiced for years. You may need to adapt these behaviors. For example, the avoidance of smoking and excessive alcohol use are important parts of an action plan for osteoporosis.

Avoid smoking. Studies show that cigarette smoking increases the rate of bone loss. Women who smoke have lower estrogen levels compared with those who don't smoke. Women smokers also

Complementary and alternative treatments

In dealing with the pain or anxiety associated with osteoporosis, perhaps you've considered complementary or alternative treatments such as acupuncture or meditation. Such therapies have become more popular as Americans seek greater control of their own health.

Complementary and alternative medicine is generally defined as treatments and health care practices that aren't widely studied or taught in medical schools, not generally used in hospitals and not usually reimbursed by health insurance companies. Many of these therapies aren't new, and some have been practiced for thousands of years. Often they emphasize a holistic approach that involves the physical, mental, emotional and spiritual aspects of health. Some complementary and alternative therapies are consistent with conventional medicine, and others aren't accepted in conventional practice.

Complementary and alternative therapies include biofeedback, guided imagery, humor, hypnosis, meditation, massage, acupuncture, homeopathy and herbal preparations.

No complementary or alternative treatment has been proven effective specifically for treating osteoporosis. However, studies indicate that biofeedback, meditation and relaxation techniques can be useful in treating chronic pain, which can occur with osteoporotic fractures. Various methods for managing chronic pain are discussed in Chapter 11.

If you have osteoporosis, be cautious about two forms of alternative medicine — chiropractic treatment and massage.

tend to undergo menopause earlier. Cigarette smokers tend to be thinner. All of these factors increase the risk of osteoporosis, and may lead to more fractures than in nonsmokers.

Avoid excessive alcohol use. This warning doesn't mean a glass of wine with meals is necessarily harmful. But studies show that drinking above moderate levels — defined as no more than two drinks a day for men and one drink a day for women — over a long period of time can hasten bone loss and reduce your body's

These can cause or aggravate spinal fractures. Talk to your doctor before trying any form of spinal manipulation.

Before using any complementary or alternative treatments, consider these suggestions:

Gather information about the treatment. Learn about the treatment from reputable sources, such as Web sites created by major medical centers, national organizations, universities or government agencies. Try to locate good evidence that the treatment is effective.

Find and evaluate treatment providers. Check your state government listings for agencies that regulate and license health care providers. Contact professional organizations for names of certified practitioners. Get advice from a trusted health care professional.

Consider treatment cost. Many complementary and alternative approaches aren't covered by health insurance. Find out exactly how much the treatment will cost.

Check your attitude. Steer a middle course between uncritical acceptance and outright rejection. Stay open to various treatments but evaluate them carefully.

Opt for a combined approach. You may choose to use complementary and alternative treatments to maintain good health and relieve some symptoms, but continue to rely on conventional medicine to treat the disease. Put greater trust in proven, effective treatments over unproven alternative ones. Tell your doctor about all of the treatments you get, both conventional and unconventional.

ability to absorb calcium. Alcohol can affect hormones that regulate calcium levels in your body and reduce the formation of new bone.

People who drink heavily are more prone to fractures because of an increased risk of falling. Bone loss can be compounded by poor nutrition because heavy drinkers often fail to eat regular, healthy meals. Chronic alcoholism can also lead to malabsorption of critical nutrients, such as calcium, magnesium and zinc. So if you do drink, try to stay at moderate levels.

Perfecting your posture

Your action plan can also include the practice of good posture, which is crucial to preventing falls and avoiding an excessively curved back. *Posture* refers to the positions of different body parts in relation to one another, whether you're standing, sitting, lying down or moving. Good posture allows your back to follow the mild S-shaped curve of the spine. It places only minimal strain on your muscles and joints and allows you to move efficiently. Good posture can help relieve the aches and pains caused by muscles, bones and ligaments that aren't in their natural positions.

For many people, poor posture is an ingrained habit. Good posture takes practice, especially if you're trying to change years of bad habits. Knowing how to sit, stand and move properly can help you avoid fractures and limit the exaggerated curvature of the spine that results from compression fractures. For more information about good posture and safe movements, see Chapter 11.

Meeting the challenge

All of the elements described in this chapter, including diet, physical activity, medications, healthy behaviors and correct posture can help you maintain bone strength and avoid fractures. Each element helps to address a different, vital aspect of your health. But no individual element is sufficient in itself to prevent or treat osteoporosis — each component works best in combination with the others.

Combined, these elements pack a stronger punch in your fight against bone loss. For example, research shows that getting enough calcium in the diet enhances the positive effects of exercise and of medication on bone density for postmenopausal women.

The following chapters provide practical suggestions for implementing your action plan and playing a more active role in your health care. This in turn will help you stay in control and may help you enjoy a more active, fulfilling life.

Chapter 8

Eating for healthy bones

L ike any living tissue, bones need nutrients to be able to grow and maintain themselves. Most nutrients aren't produced by the body and must be provided by food. A lack of nutrients in your diet can lead to stunted growth, weaker bones and disease. Expressed in positive terms, the better your diet, the stronger your bones and the less chance you have of developing osteoporosis.

A varied diet with the right balance of calories, vitamins and minerals is the starting point for healthy bones. To prevent and treat osteoporosis, you need to pay particular attention to getting enough of the mineral calcium and vitamin D.

The best way to boost your calcium intake is by choosing foods high in calcium content. If you drink milk, you're off to a great start. Milk is often fortified with vitamin D. Finding ways to incorporate other high-calcium foods into your diet is a fun, healthy and tasty experience.

The previous chapter talked about diet in the context of various factors you'll need to incorporate into an action plan for osteoporosis. This chapter discusses the basics of good nutrition as well as practical ways to increase your calcium intake — where to find it, how to get more of it, calcium-rich recipes, calcium supplements and more. Eating is a pleasure as well as a necessity, so enjoy yourself with this part of your action plan.

Good nutrition in a nutshell

Variety is not just the spice of life, it's the basis of a healthy diet. No single food provides all of the nutrients your body needs. Eating a variety of foods ensures you'll get the vitamins, minerals, proteins, carbohydrates and fiber that optimize nutrition, good health and a healthy weight.

Meal planning and preparation doesn't have to be complicated. One simple approach is to follow national nutrition guidelines found in the Dietary Guidelines for Americans, from the U.S. Department of Agriculture. These guidelines promote variety, balance and moderation in your food choices. They incorporate the best judgment of nutrition professionals based on current knowledge about how diet influences health and helps prevent disease. The key recommendations are summarized as follows:

- Eat more fruits, vegetables and grains.
- Reduce fat and cholesterol.
- Limit sugar, salt and phosphate additives.
- Limit consumption of alcohol and caffeine.

Eat more fruits, vegetables and grains

Choose a variety of vegetables, fruits and grains for your daily meals. These foods are generally lower in calories and fat, so you have fewer worries about how much to eat. They're high in fiber, essential vitamins and minerals, and phytochemicals, substances that may help protect against a variety of diseases, including osteoporosis. Studies show that higher intake of fruits and vegetables — and lower intake of protein from meat sources — leads to improved bone health.

Aim to eat four or more servings of vegetables and three or more servings of fruit each day. It's best if they are fresh and not processed. Because different fruits and vegetables provide different nutrients, variety is vital. Depending on your calorie level, eat four to eight servings of grains — cereal, bread, rice and pasta — each day. Choose whole grains when possible because they contain more nutrients and fiber than refined grains do. You may be eating some whole grains without realizing it, such as oatmeal and popcorn.

How many calories do you need?

The Dietary Guidelines for Americans suggest the following daily calorie amounts:

- Children ages 2 to 6, most women, older adults: about 1,600
- Older children, teen girls, active women, most men: about 2,200
- Teen boys, active men: about 2,800

If you're trying to lose weight, the daily calorie goal for most men will generally be 1,400 to 1,800, and for most women, about 1,200 to 1,600.

Reduce fat and cholesterol

You need some fat in your diet in order for your body to function properly. But too much fat or the wrong type of fat can have a negative impact on your health. For example, saturated fat increases your risk of coronary artery disease by raising blood cholesterol. Animal foods such as meat and dairy products contain varying amounts of saturated fat and cholesterol.

Aim for a total fat intake of no more than 30 percent of the calories you consume each day, with 10 percent or less coming from saturated fat. Try to keep your daily cholesterol intake to less than 300 milligrams (mg). Foods high in saturated fats include high-fat dairy products, meat and foods made from chocolate, lard, solid shortenings, palm oil and coconut oil. Concentrated sources of cholesterol include egg yolks and organ meats such as liver.

For bone — and heart — health, make sure that your meat choices are lean and limit the total amount of meat to 5 or 6 ounces daily. Try to choose fat-free or low-fat milk, low-fat cheese and fat-free or low-fat yogurt. Choose foods that contain monosaturated fats, such as olive oil or canola oil.

Limit sugar, salt and phosphate additives

Foods containing sugars that are added during processing generally provide a lot of calories but few vitamins, minerals and other nutrients. For these reasons, dietary guidelines often recommend that you limit foods and beverages containing added sugars.

In the United States, the No. 1 source of added sugar in the diet is soft drinks. In the past two decades, the percentage of people in the United States consuming soft drinks increased by 32 percent, and the percentage of those drinking milk decreased by 18 percent. According to one study, children who regularly chose soft drinks over milk or juice weren't likely to meet daily recommendations for the nutrients that they need for normal growth and development.

Most Americans also consume too much salt (sodium chloride). The recommended daily amount is 2,400 milligrams (mg), which is equivalent to about 1 teaspoon of salt. Most of the salt you eat is found in processed foods. Studies show that high levels of sodium are associated with high blood pressure. In addition, a high salt intake increases the amount of calcium you excrete.

Phosphorus, in the form of phosphates, is used as an additive in many processed foods, such as hot dogs, chicken nuggets, chips, processed cheeses and spreads, instant gravies, sauces, fillings and puddings and frozen products that are breaded. Too much phosphorus in your diet can interfere with how much calcium is absorbed through your small intestine.

To limit your intake of sugar, salt and phosphate additives, choose and prepare your foods carefully. Check the labels on processed foods you buy at the grocery store. Inquire about the details of food content at fast-food establishments. When preparing meals, use herbs, spices and fruits to flavor food.

Limit consumption of alcohol and caffeine

Alcoholic beverages supply calories but few nutrients. They can be harmful for many reasons when consumed in excess, and some people shouldn't drink alcohol at all. If you drink alcoholic beverages, do so in moderation. Consuming more than one to two drinks a day can hasten bone loss and reduce your body's ability to absorb calcium. Drink alcohol with meals to slow its absorption. Women planning to be or already pregnant should not drink at all.

Caffeine can reduce calcium absorption slightly, but much of the potentially harmful effect is due to caffeinated beverages too often being substituted for healthier drinks, such as milk. Moderate caffeine consumption — about two to three cups of coffee a day —

won't harm you as long as your diet contains adequate calcium. You can offset calcium loss owing to coffee drinking by adding a tablespoon or two of milk to each cup.

Calcium in your diet

You know that calcium is a nutrition superstar when it comes to bone health. But if you're like most Americans, you may not be getting enough calcium every day. The typical American diet provides less than 600 mg of calcium a day, but the recommended daily intake for most adults ranges from 1,000 to 1,200 mg or more. (See Chapter 7 for the specific calcium requirements.)

The obvious way to increase your calcium intake is to include in your meals foods that are high in calcium. Milk and other dairy products, such as yogurt and cheese, are the richest sources of calcium. You can choose fat-free and low-fat varieties that contain the same amount of calcium as higher-fat products. Milk is also fortified with vitamin D and supplies the daily requirement of this nutrient in one serving. Dairy products aren't the only foods that are rich in calcium. Other sources are listed in "Food sources of calcium" on pages 108 to 109.

In addition, many foods have calcium added to them. Calcium-fortified products include breakfast cereals, breads, pasta, rice, pancake and waffle mixes, juices, bottled water, soy beverages and products such as margarine. Check the product label to determine the calcium content.

It's easier to meet calcium requirements with dairy products than with other foods. For example, 1 cup of milk contains the same amount of calcium as about 3 to 4 cups of broccoli. If you can't or choose not to eat dairy products, you may have to work a little harder to make sure you get enough calcium. If you have difficulty digesting milk, you can meet your calcium needs by consuming lactose-free milk products and calcium-fortified foods or by taking a supplement. (See "Lactose intolerance" on page 114.)

Studies suggest that eating food sources of calcium is better for you than calcium supplements because the foods contain other

Assessing your calcium intake

Are you getting enough calcium? A diet without dairy products or calcium-rich foods generally provides about 200 to 300 milligrams (mg) of calcium a day. To calculate your daily calcium intake, you may assume you get about 300 mg from these nondairy sources. Add 300 mg for each dairy product serving you consume, which is the equivalent of about 1 cup of milk, yogurt or calcium-fortified juice or 2 ounces of hard cheese. Then add the amount from any supplements you take.

Let's take a look at the calcium intake for a woman whose only dairy product for the day is milk with her cereal but who also takes a calcium supplement:

Nondairy sources	300 mg
Dairy servings (½ cup milk)	150 mg
One calcium supplement	600 mg
Total calcium	1,050 mg

important nutrients as well. For example, milk also provides protein, vitamins A, D and B-12, magnesium, riboflavin, potassium and zinc. Dietary calcium may reduce the risk of high blood pressure and kidney stones, but calcium supplements don't have this effect.

Tips for increasing your calcium intake

Now that you know which foods are high in calcium, work on finding ways to make these foods part of your daily diet. Try to eat at least one serving of a calcium-rich food at each meal. Three servings a day can provide as much as 900 mg of calcium toward your daily need for 1,000 to 1,200 mg. To get started and get inspired, consider the following tips:

- Add 1 ounce — about a slice or two — of Swiss cheese to your sandwich for an extra 270 mg of calcium.
- Make soup with low-fat milk instead of water. A 2-cup portion of soup will provide at least 300 mg of calcium.

- Prepare instant oatmeal with low-fat milk instead of water —
$\frac{1}{2}$ cup of low-fat milk added to a packet of oatmeal provides at
least 150 mg of calcium. Fortified instant oats provide another
160 mg.
- Instead of the same old sour cream dip, which has minimal
calcium and lots of fat, dip vegetables and fruit into fat-free
yogurt. Most varieties of plain yogurt has at least 450 mg of
calcium per cup.
- Like Southern-style foods? One cup of each of the following
has about 150 to 200 mg of calcium: cooked greens (turnip,
collard, kale, beet or spinach), okra, black-eyed peas and white
beans. A baking powder biscuit has about 150 mg of calcium.
- Fortify a smoothie by substituting $\frac{1}{2}$ cup of low-fat milk or
yogurt for water or using $\frac{1}{2}$ cup of calcium-fortified orange
juice instead of plain juice. This adds 150 to 200 mg of calcium.
You may also mix in a tablespoon of malt powder (60 mg of
calcium) or dark molasses (170 mg of calcium).
- Gourmet treatment can add a calcium punch to plain foods.
Serve eggs or fish on a one-cup bed of cooked spinach a la
Florentine for about 240 mg of calcium. Or add 50 mg of calcium when you garnish vegetables or fish amandine with 3
tablespoons of slivered almonds.
- Like Asian foods? Think soy. Many soy foods are a great
source of calcium. These include *edamame*, the Japanese word
for "green soybeans", which is commonly found in the super-
market with other frozen vegetables. One cup has about 260
mg of calcium. Firm tofu can be used in place of meat, poultry
or fish in a stir-fry, with 860 mg of calcium per $\frac{1}{2}$ cup. Snack
on soy nuts, which are dried soybeans. One-third cup has
about 80 mg of calcium.
- When cooking, remember not to add milk to hot ingredients
because milk scorches easily. Instead, add hot ingredients
gradually to the milk and then bring the whole mixture up to
temperature. Most recipes containing milk can also be cooked
without scorching in the microwave or in a double boiler.
When using ingredients that are high in acid, prevent curdling
by adding them to the milk gradually rather than vice versa.

Food sources of calcium

Foods	Amount	Calories	Calcium (milligrams)
Dairy			
Yogurt, plain, low-fat	1 cup	140	485
Yogurt, fruited, low-fat	1 cup	250	340-370
Milk, whole	1 cup	150	300
Milk, low-fat (2 percent)	1 cup	120	300
Milk, skim	1 cup	90	300
Milk, fat-free, dry powder	⅓ cup	90	280
Yogurt, frozen, low-fat	1 cup	220	205
Pudding, with skim milk	½ cup	105	150
Ice cream (10-percent fat)	½ cup	130	90
Ice milk	½ cup	90	90
Cheese			
Ricotta, part skim milk	1 cup	339	669
Swiss	1 ounce	110	270
Cheddar	1 ounce	115	205
Mozzarella, part skim milk	1 ounce	80	205
American, processed	1 ounce	90	160
Cottage, low-fat (from 2-percent milk)	1 cup	200	150
Cottage, regular from whole milk	1 cup	230	135
Cottage, fat-free	1 cup	123	45
Fish and shellfish			
Sardines, canned, with bones	3 ounces (6 sardines)	177	325
Salmon, canned, with bones	3 ounces	120	180
Herring, pickled	3 ounces	220	65
Shrimp	3 ounces	84	33
Fruit			
Orange juice, calcium fortified	1 cup	105	300
Papaya	1 medium	120	70
Orange	1 medium	70	60

Foods	Amount	Calories	Calcium (milligrams)
Vegetables			
Rhubarb (sweetened, cooked or frozen)	½ cup	140	175
Soybeans (cooked)	½ cup	125	130
Spinach (fresh, cooked)	½ cup	20	120
Collard, mustard greens	½ cup	25	115
Black-eyed peas, cow peas	½ cup	80	105
Turnip greens (fresh, cooked)	½ cup	15	100
Kale (frozen, cooked)	½ cup	20	90
Okra (fresh)	½ cup	25	90
Chinese cabbage (boiled)	½ cup	10	80
Beans, great northern, white (dried or cooked)	½ cup	105-125	60-80
Swiss chard (boiled)	½ cup	20	50
Broccoli (frozen, cooked)	½ cup	20	35
Broccoli (fresh, cooked)	½ cup	22	35
Carrots	½ cup	25	16
Other foods			
Soy milk, calcium fortified	1 cup	80	250
Pizza with cheese	1 slice	280	232
Cereal, fortified	Check label on cereal box		200-300
Macaroni and cheese	1 cup	430	200
Tomato soup, with milk	1 cup	160	160
Dark molasses	1 tablespoon	40	140
Almonds, oil roasted	1 ounce (about 20)	170	80
Tofu (soybean curd), prepared with calcium	½ cup	90-180	40-860
Hummus	½ cup	205	40
Peanuts, oil roasted	1 ounce	165	25
Sunflower seeds	1 ounce	175	15
Cashews, oil roasted	1 ounce	165	10

Bone-healthy menus and recipes

Below are two sample menus developed by Mayo Clinic dietitians that provide the recommended amount of daily calcium. The menus emphasize whole grains, vegetables, fruits and low-fat dairy products. This variety helps provide plentiful amounts of calcium and other nutrients. Each day's menu is based on a diet of 2,000 calories, with no more than 30 percent of the calories coming from fat. Sodium is limited to less than 2,400 mg a day. "Bone" appetit!

Menu 1

Breakfast
- 1 cup whole-wheat flakes cereal, topped with half a peach
- 2 slices whole-grain toast
- 1 teaspoon soft margarine
- 1 cup skim milk

Lunch
- Turkey sandwich a la Mediterranean: 1 ounce turkey, 1 ounce part-skim mozzarella cheese, ½ sliced tomato and 2 tablespoons pesto sauce on 2 slices whole-wheat bread
- 1 fresh apple
- 1 cup fresh vegetables, for example, raw baby carrots, celery sticks and broccoli florets
- 6 ounces cranberry juice

Dinner
- 4 ounces grilled salmon steak with lemon pepper
- ½ cup (3 small) roasted new potatoes
- Spinach with feta cheese and almonds (See page 115)
- 1 whole-wheat roll
- 1 tablespoon honey
- 1 cup skim milk

Snack (anytime)
- 1 ounce (¼ cup) unsalted pretzels

Menu 1 nutritional analysis

Food servings		Nutrient content per menu	
Grain/carbohydrate	9	Calories	1,700
Fruits	3	Fat (grams, or g)	42
Vegetables	3	Saturated fat (g)	10
Protein/dairy	6	Cholesterol (mg)	115
Fats	2	Sodium (mg)	1,500
Sweets	1	Calcium (mg)	1,300

Menu 2

Breakfast

- Omelet: 1 egg, 2 egg whites, 1½ ounces low-fat cheddar cheese, ¼ cup chopped onion, ¼ cup chopped tomato
- 1 medium cornmeal muffin
- 2 teaspoons fruit spread
- 6 ounces calcium-fortified orange juice
- Decaffeinated coffee

Lunch

- Wild rice soup (see page 112)
- 12 wheat crackers
- Sliced tomato with cucumbers, sprinkled with dill
- ¾ cup blueberries
- 1 cup fat-free yogurt
- Herbal tea or any other calorie-free beverage

Dinner

- Grilled chicken and vegetable kebabs: Marinate chicken in pineapple juice. Skewer and grill chicken pieces, bell peppers, cherry tomatoes and pineapple chunks.
- 1 cup yolkless egg noodles, tossed with 1 teaspoon olive oil and sprinkled with caraway seeds
- Spring greens with orange segments and light vinaigrette
- Green tea or any other calorie-free beverage

Bone-healthy menus and recipes

Snack (anytime)

- 2 cups unsalted air-popped popcorn
- Sparkling water with twist of lime

Menu 2 nutritional analysis

Food servings		Nutrient content per menu	
Grain/carbohydrate	6	Calories	1,650
Fruits	4	Fat (g)	45
Vegetables	4	Saturated fat (g)	13
Protein/dairy	5	Cholesterol (mg)	260
Fats	2	Sodium (mg)	1,050
Sweets	1	Calcium (mg)	1,160

Recipes

Wild rice soup
Serves 6 (about 1½ cups per serving)

- 1 tablespoon margarine
- ½ cup diced onion
- 1 cup diced celery
- ⅔ cup sliced mushrooms
- ½ cup cubed turkey
- ¼ cup flour
- 4 cups reduced-sodium chicken broth
- ¼ cup fat-free dry milk
- ½ cup skim milk
- 1½ cups cooked wild rice
- Cracked black pepper to taste

Saute onions, celery, mushrooms and turkey in margarine. Add flour and stir well. Add chicken broth, dry milk and skim milk, stirring constantly. Add cooked wild rice. Simmer. Season with cracked black pepper. Serve.

Wild rice soup nutritional analysis

Food servings	Nutrient content per serving
Grain/carbohydrate...... ½	Calories 150
Protein/dairy 1½	Fat (g) 4
	Saturated fat (g) 1
	Cholesterol (mg)........ 9
	Sodium (mg).......... 200
	Calcium (mg) 80

Chocolate ricotta mousse

Serves 6 (generous ½-cup portions)

• 3 ounces unsweetened chocolate, melted
• 1 pound ricotta cheese
• 1 teaspoon vanilla
• ⅓ cup honey

Blend melted chocolate, ricotta cheese, vanilla and honey in a blender or food processor until very smooth. Pour mixture into dessert cups and chill. To serve, garnish each serving with a fresh ripe strawberry, a few raspberries or an orange or kiwi slice.

Chocolate ricotta mousse nutritional analysis

Food servings	Nutrient content per serving
Protein/dairy............ 2	Calories 230
Fats 2	Fat (g) 8
	Saturated fat (g) 4
	Cholesterol (mg)........ 24
	Sodium (mg).......... 105
	Calcium (mg) 230

Bone-healthy menus and recipes

Tropical smoothie

Serves 4

- 1 cup vanilla yogurt
- 1 cup calcium-fortified orange juice
- 1 banana
- ½ cup crushed unsweetened pineapple

Place all ingredients into a blender. Blend until smooth and serve. To make a thicker, chilly smoothie, freeze the banana and pineapple before blending.

Tropical smoothie nutritional analysis

Food servings	Nutrient content per serving
Fruits. 1	Calories 110
Protein/dairy. 1	Fat (g) . . . . trace
	Saturated fat (g) . . . . . . trace
	Cholesterol (mg). . . . . . trace
	Sodium (mg). 35
	Calcium (mg). 115

Lactose intolerance

Does milk or ice cream upset your stomach sometimes? You may have lactose intolerance — the inability to fully digest the sugar in milk (lactose) and other dairy products. Signs and symptoms of lactose intolerance may include bloating, cramping, gas, diarrhea and nausea. Discomfort usually begins 30 minutes to 2 hours after ingesting foods that contain lactose.

If you're lactose intolerant, you still need calcium. And you probably don't need to forgo dairy products completely. Many people with lactose intolerance can comfortably digest a glass of milk with a meal. And people who can't tolerate milk often have no problem with hard cheeses, yogurt and lactose-reduced milk. If you prefer not to consume dairy products, you can meet your daily calcium needs with calcium-fortified foods and calcium supplements.

Spinach with feta cheese and almonds

Serves 6 (generous ½-cup portions)

- ¼ cup slivered almonds
- 1 teaspoon extra-virgin olive oil
- 1 large clove garlic, chopped
- 4 scallions or green garden onions with tops, chopped
- 1½ pounds spinach, stems removed and well washed in several changes of cold water
- A small amount of water
- Freshly ground black pepper
- 4 ounces crumbled feta cheese, at room temperature
- Lemon wedges

Toast slivered almonds in a saute pan over medium heat until slightly browned and fragrant. Put aside to cool. In the same pan, heat oil, add garlic and scallions and cook gently for 15 to 20 seconds, being careful not to let the garlic brown. Add spinach and a bit of water. Cover and cook for about 1 minute. The spinach will wilt rapidly. Remove from heat and top with black pepper, feta cheese crumbles and toasted almonds. Serve immediately, garnished with lemon wedges.

Spinach with feta cheese and almonds nutritional analysis

Food servings		Nutrient content per serving	
Protein/dairy	1	Calories	115
Fats	1	Fat (g)	7
		Saturated fat (g)	2
		Cholesterol (mg)	15
		Sodium (mg)	300
		Calcium (mg)	225

Calcium supplements

If you aren't getting enough calcium in your diet, you may need a calcium supplement to make up for what you're lacking. A supplement is often recommended for postmenopausal women because calcium supplementation can reduce the rate of bone loss.

Types

Choosing a calcium supplement can be confusing. Several different calcium compounds are used in supplements. The different compounds contain varying amounts of what's known as elemental calcium — the actual amount of calcium that's available to your body. Because the recommended daily amounts of calcium are given in terms of elemental calcium, you'll need to read the package labels carefully. Adding a zero to the "percent daily value" for calcium listed on the label will give the milligrams of elemental calcium.

Calcium carbonate, calcium citrate and calcium phosphate are the most common compounds. They're available as pills, capsules, effervescents, candy and chewable tablets. To choose, consider your own preferences and which supplement best agrees with you.

Calcium carbonate. This is the least expensive and most commonly used compound. Calcium carbonate may cause constipation. It works best when taken with meals.

Chewable antacids such as Rolaids and Tums contain high levels of calcium carbonate. Check the labels so that you know how much elemental calcium you're getting. Along with calcium carbonate, Viactiv Calcium Chews contain vitamins D and K to help increase calcium absorption. One note of caution: If you're also taking medications to thin your blood, such as warfarin (Coumadin), talk to your doctor before taking Viactiv. Because vitamin K affects blood clotting, your dose of blood thinner may need to be adjusted.

Calcium citrate. This compound is the most easily absorbed and doesn't have to be taken with meals. It's also less concentrated than calcium carbonate, so you may need to take at least twice as many tablets to reach the recommended amount.

Calcium phosphate. This compound also requires multiple doses but is least likely to cause constipation.

Calcium and vitamin D content of common supplements

Product	Elemental calcium per tablet (mg)	Vitamin D (international units or IU)	Other ingredients
Calcium carbonate			
Alka-Mints	340	0	
Caltrate 600 + D	600	200	
Caltrate 600 Plus	600	200	Zinc, copper, magnesium
Caltrate 600 + Soy	600	200	25 mg soy isoflavones
Centrum Silver	200	400	Multivitamin
Mylanta Gelcaps	220	0	125 mg magnesium
Mylanta Maximum Strength	280	0	300 mg magnesium
One-A-Day Calcium Plus	500	100	50 mg magnesium
Os-Cal 500 + D	500	200	Oyster shell powder
Os-Cal Ultra 600	600	200	Other vitamins and minerals
Rolaids	220	0	
Rolaids Extra Strength	270	0	
Tums	200	0	
Tums Ultra	400	0	
Viactiv	500	100	40 mg vitamin K
Calcium citrate			
Citracal	200	0	
Citracal + D	315	200	
GNC A-Z Calcium Citrate Plus	200	25	100 mg magnesium
Calcium phosphate			
Posture-D	600	125	266 mg phosphorus

Milk myths

Got milk? No way, say some people. Like many foods, milk has its critics. They express concerns about the health and safety of milk and other dairy products. Here are some misconceptions about milk:

It makes you fat. To limit fat and calorie intake, some people needlessly rule out all dairy products. But regular consumption of low-fat versions of milk, yogurt and cheese may actually help control body fat. A recent study showed that milk fat was not associated with the harmful effects usually associated with other fats. In fact, people with high milk intakes had smaller waistlines and weighed less than those who avoided dairy products. Another study showed that young women who consumed calcium from dairy foods experienced greater weight loss benefits than did those who used nondairy sources or supplements.

It weakens bones. Sound scientific research has shown that milk and dairy products are good sources of nutrients that are vital for strong bones. For example, several randomized, controlled clinical trials — the gold standard of medical research — that used dairy products all showed significantly positive effects on bone health.

Getting the most out of calcium supplements

When you take a calcium supplement, you want to make sure that your body absorbs as much of the mineral as it can. The following tips will help you maximize absorption and reduce the risks of unpleasant side effects, such as constipation and gas.

- Read supplement labels carefully. Different calcium supplements have different amounts of elemental calcium. For example, although a label advertises 1,250 mg of calcium carbonate, the supplement may actually contain only 500 mg of elemental calcium. Also pay attention to the serving size. The label may list 1,000 mg of elemental calcium in each serving, but the serving may consist of three tablets.
- Taking a large amount of calcium at one time reduces how much calcium is absorbed. You can increase absorption by tak-

It causes allergies. Milk allergies are usually a reaction to certain components in milk, such as the protein casein (KA-seen). Such allergies are uncommon. About 1 percent to 3 percent of children experience allergies to cow's milk, and they usually outgrow this by age 3. In adults, milk allergies are even rarer. On the other hand, lactose intolerance is fairly common, but most people with this intolerance can consume small amounts of milk or dairy products without experiencing symptoms. (See "Lactose intolerance" on page 114.)

It's full of antibiotics and hormones. The use of antibiotics and hormones in animal foods is controversial. However, even critics have found no residue in milk. The Food and Drug Administration (FDA) has approved the use of bovine somatotropin (bST) to promote milk production in dairy cattle. This hormone occurs naturally in milk and is biologically inactive in humans. Even so, you can buy milk made from cows not given bST — the packages are labeled to reflect this.

Many people avoid milk and dairy products because of such misconceptions. Unfortunately, they're depriving themselves of foods they may enjoy and that provide important nutrients, especially calcium.

ing smaller amounts of calcium several times a day. Try to limit a dose to no more than 500 mg of elemental calcium.

- Take your calcium supplements with meals or on a full stomach. This helps increase absorption.
- Look for the letters *USP* on the package label. These initials stand for U.S. Pharmacopeia, the government organization that sets standards for how well a supplement dissolves. In general, stick to brand names with proven reliability — which usually carry the USP designation — or ask your pharmacist to recommend a supplement.
- Avoid "natural" calcium preparations that contain oyster shell, bone meal or dolomite. These supplements may be contaminated with lead, aluminum or other toxic substances that can have harmful effects.

- If you often forget to take your supplement, use a 7-day pill-box to help you keep track of your doses.
- Don't take more than 2,500 mg of calcium a day.

Side effects

Calcium supplements may cause gas, bloating and constipation in some people. To avoid such side effects, drink at least six to eight glasses of water daily, exercise and make sure to eat plenty of vegetables, fruits and whole grains. If you develop any symptoms with one type of calcium supplement, switch to a different preparation. For example, try switching from calcium carbonate to calcium citrate, which is less likely to cause constipation.

If you have a history of kidney stones, you should talk to your doctor before taking any calcium supplement. A high calcium intake, primarily through supplements, may also increase your risk of prostate cancer.

Chapter 9

Staying active

L ike the rest of your body, your bones thrive on movement. Physical activity increases bone mass during childhood, helps you maintain bone density as a young adult and can help offset bone loss as you age. Exercise also helps your posture and improves your balance, which in turn reduces the risk of falls. Beyond the bone benefits, physical activity keeps you healthy and strong and can give you more energy.

This chapter guides you on the path to a more active life. The exercises described in the following pages are designed to strengthen your bones while minimizing your risk of fractures. No matter what your age or condition, physical activity can be a simple, pleasurable part of your day.

Putting theory into practice

You may have always known that exercise is good for you, but in the past you didn't have the time or the energy or the right equipment. Maybe you found exercise boring, or you were afraid of getting injured. In fact, 60 percent of the U.S. population doesn't exercise. Less than one-fourth of Americans are regularly active, and more than half of those who start exercising quit within 6 months.

If you're at risk of osteoporosis or already have it, it's even more important to find ways to fit physical activity into your life. You may be reluctant to exercise because of concerns about injury or pain. But avoiding physical activity only aggravates bone loss and puts the skeleton in greater jeopardy. Your goal will be to make physical activity a routine part of your day.

Physical activity doesn't have to be a tedious chore requiring long hours at the gym, fancy workout clothes or specialized equipment. Routine tasks can be just as important as formal exercise sessions. *Exercise* is a structured, planned approach that's often measured or timed, such as when you regularly do 15 stretches or walk briskly for 30 minutes. *Activity* refers to almost every motion of your body as you go about performing daily tasks and living your life — including exercise. Spending a part of each day straightening up the house, shopping, mowing the lawn, walking the dog or gardening can contribute to bone strength if done on a regular basis.

Although the activities of daily living are vital to any action plan for osteoporosis, the needs and capabilities of one person are quite different from those of another. This type of activity will need to be assessed individually by you and your doctor.

This chapter focuses on a simple exercise program to supplement the regular activities in your day. It's hoped that a few general rules and tips will allow almost anyone, regardless of his or her specific circumstance, to establish a safe exercise routine. Several of the exercises described in this chapter may appeal to you and be included in your routine, but many other exercises would be suitable choices too.

Getting started

If you're trying to prevent or treat osteoporosis, the types of activities and exercises you choose to do will be based on your goals, overall health status, degree of bone loss and what you enjoy doing. You may want to avoid some exercises and movements that could cause more damage to your bones. What's appropriate for one individual may not help another. Your doctor can help you determine what exercises will do you the most good and how intensely to do them.

The important thing is to participate safely in *some* activity in a regular and sustained manner. Any safe exercise is better than no exercise. And the best bet is to choose enjoyable exercises that you're likely to stay with for the long haul.

Often a combination of different exercises is recommended to help prevent or treat osteoporosis. These include weight-bearing exercises, resistance exercises and back-strengthening exercises.

Consult the specialists

If you have osteoporosis, talk to your doctor before starting an exercise program. For one thing, a doctor can assess your overall health status and family medical history, such as whether you or anyone in your family has or had cardiovascular disease or high blood pressure. Be aware that some medications, especially tranquilizers and those that help you sleep, can affect the way your body reacts to exercise. Ask your doctor about how your medications may affect your exercise plan.

You may also want to consult a physical therapist or exercise specialist about appropriate exercise routines, including warm-up and cool-down periods. A physical therapist can also demonstrate proper body mechanics, safe methods for stretching and strengthening muscles and proper use of the equipment you use. Some hospitals and fitness centers offer special exercise classes for people with osteoporosis.

Assess your fitness level

Although some conditions, including osteoporosis, may prevent you from doing certain activities, almost everyone can participate in some form of exercise. It's helpful to have a realistic appraisal of your fitness level as you plan your routine.

If you can easily do all of your normal daily activities at a reasonable pace without becoming breathless or dizzy, breaking into a sweat or having chest pain, you're probably fit enough for a sample exercise program. But keep in mind that other components of fitness, such as flexibility and muscle strength, also are important.

Signs of not being fit (deconditioning) include feeling tired most of the time, being unable to keep up with the pace of others your age, avoiding activities because you know you'll tire quickly, and becoming short of breath or fatigued after walking a short distance.

If you've been inactive or in a weakened condition or you have low bone density, don't expect to be able to run 3 miles and lift heavy weights. And don't plan to work out 2 hours a day, 365 days a year. Begin with short amounts of physical exercise — perhaps no more than 5 to 10 minutes. If all goes well, begin to gradually increase your activity. Try to keep physical exertion at a level you can safely and comfortably perform.

Set your goals

Setting goals is a good way to get motivated and stick with your exercise program. Try to make your goals realistic and achievable. It's always encouraging to see or feel some results as you exercise. On the other hand, setting your goals too high may lead to disillusionment and failure.

If you have osteoporosis, your goals for being physically active may be associated with:

- Increasing your ability to carry out daily tasks and activities
- Maintaining or improving your posture and balance
- Relieving or lessening pain
- Preventing falls and fracture
- Increasing your sense of well-being

If you have chronic pain, your goals in exercising may be to lessen your pain and increase your ability to move. After consulting with your doctor or physical therapist, you may come up with a list of several gentle stretches to try. Perhaps your initial goal will be to do a certain number of stretches each day for a week. At the end of the week, note whether your pain has lessened and whether you're able to move a bit more easily. If so, consider increasing your activity — adding a short walk to your day or increasing the number of stretching exercises you do. If you're not feeling better, talk to your doctor about other possible exercises.

If your overall goal is to improve your posture, perhaps start with a few balance and posture exercises every other day. Or maybe your goal is to walk briskly for 30 minutes 4 days a week. Start with 10 to 15 minutes and build from there.

It's important to monitor your activity and adapt what you do so that it serves you best. You might want to keep an exercise diary to chart your progress.

Avoid risky movements

If you have low bone density or already have osteoporosis, a few precautions are necessary when you exercise or perform regular activities. Certain movements may be dangerous because of the stress they put on the spine. You may not be able to avoid these movements altogether, so use caution and be sure to practice good posture and body mechanics when doing them. Pay attention to how you move.

Forward bending. Avoid activities and exercises that involve bending forward because they increase the risk of compression fractures of your vertebrae. Try not to let your back bend forward as you make the bed, tie your shoes, pull weeds, reach down to pick up something from the floor and other such activities. Instead, keep your back straight as you bend at the knees to lower your body. Forward bending of the torso is especially dangerous if you're carrying anything, as when you take a heavy pan out of the oven or set a bag of groceries on the floor.

Heavy lifting. Avoid heavy lifting, which may include loads of laundry, bags of groceries or exercise weights. This lifting will increase the stress on your vertebrae. If you must lift a heavy object, carry it close to your body. Be careful about opening windows or a garage door.

Twisting. Twisting movements can place unusual force on the spine. When you're driving, use your side mirrors for backing up and parking so that you avoid twisting to look through the rear window. Golfing and bowling are two common sports that involve twisting and may be harmful. Talk to your doctor or physical therapist about whether you can safely participate in these sports.

Reaching overhead. Reaching above your shoulders, as when you reach for something in a kitchen cupboard, isn't recommended for people with severe stooped posture (kyphosis).

Danger signs during exercise

No matter what exercise you're doing, stop and seek immediate care if you experience any of these warning signs:

- Tightness in your chest
- Severe shortness of breath
- Chest pain or pain in your arms or jaw, especially on the left side
- Heart palpitations
- Dizziness, faintness or feeling sick to your stomach

High-impact activities. Activities that involve jarring movements, sudden stops and starts, and abrupt weight shifts put too much stress on the spine and can lead to falls and knee injuries in older adults. Such activities include jogging, running, soccer, racket sports, volleyball and basketball.

Do it!

A big challenge many people face is finding the motivation to stick with an exercise program. Make a firm commitment to being active. This doesn't mean you won't have setbacks or occasionally need to take breaks. The key is to keep going even after an occasional lay-off. As you get started, consider these tips:

- Start slowly. Don't jump into an intense exercise program right away if you haven't been regularly active. Instead, focus on small amounts of activity and gradually work up to more strenuous exercise.
- Schedule exercise into your day as you would an important errand or social event. But don't be rigid about sticking to your schedule if you don't feel up to it. If you're very tired or under the weather, take a day or two off.
- Pace yourself. If you're unable to converse while exercising, you're probably working too hard.
- Listen to your body. You may feel some muscle soreness and discomfort as you begin exercising, but this shouldn't be painful and shouldn't last more than 24 to 48 hours. If pain persists, you may be working too hard and need to ease up.

Exercises for osteoporosis

Three types of exercise are often recommended for people with osteoporosis: back-strengthening exercise, weight-bearing exercise and resistance exercise. Doing a little of each in a structured program can help you to keep your bones strong and maintain good posture. Remember that physical exercise doesn't have to be strenuous or high impact to be effective.

Warming up and cooling down

It's important to allow time for warming up before any physical exercise and cooling down afterward. Warming up gradually increases your heart rate, and it limbers up your muscles, which reduces your risk of injury.

To warm up, walk slowly, then increase your pace gradually. Or begin an activity, such as bicycling or swimming, at a slower pace than what you're accustomed to until you feel loose.

End each exercise session by walking slowly or by continuing to do the activity at a slower pace. It's also a good time to stretch the muscles you used during your exercise.

Weight-bearing exercise

Weight-bearing exercises have nothing to do with weightlifting equipment. They're done on your feet with the bones of your lower body supporting your own weight. These activities help slow mineral loss in the bones of your legs, hips and lower spine.

Many young adults build bone mass through their participation in high-impact activities, which places greater loads on their bones. High-impact activities include jogging, soccer, basketball, volleyball, racket sports, gymnastics, dance and figure skating.

Older adults or people with low bone density should take precautions against too much impact and avoid activities that involve a high risk of falling. Low-impact activities such as walking will place less stress on their more fragile bones. Someone in a frail condition may opt for weight-supported exercises — as opposed to weight-bearing exercises. Weight-supported exercises include swimming, floor exercises or cycling on a stationary bike.

Low-impact weight-bearing activities

Any of the following activities would generally be a safe, invigorating choice for someone with osteoporosis:

- Walking
- Treadmill walking
- Using a cross-country ski machine
- Using a stair-climbing machine
- Doing water aerobics
- Deep-water walking
- Doing low-impact aerobics
- Cycling outdoors
- Light gardening

Source: National Osteoporosis Foundation, 2000

Remember that weight bearing is all about being on your feet. The most important thing is to choose exercises that you enjoy. Because walking improves your balance and coordination, it's also one of the best exercises for reducing your risk of falls. Don't forget your warm-up and cool-down periods.

Take a brisk walk around the block with a neighbor or walk on a treadmill while watching television. If you don't use walking as a form of regular exercise, you can still get benefits by fitting in short walks whenever possible. Make your walks more fun by bringing a friend or your spouse. On poor-weather days, consider indoor walking at a mall or a health club.

Aerobic benefits. Weight-bearing exercises also provide aerobic benefits. Aerobic activities increase your breathing and heart rates, which improve the health of your heart, lungs and circulatory system. This gives you more stamina and endurance, which make it easier to do whatever you need to do, whether it's cleaning the house or climbing the bleachers at your granddaughter's basketball game.

Even if your physician advises you to avoid weight-bearing exercises, you can still gain aerobic benefits from low- or no-impact exercises, such as swimming, water exercises and indoor cycling.

Walking: An ideal exercise

Walking is considered a safe, simple, cost-free exercise that causes minimal jarring to your bones. It requires no special equipment, lessons, other participants or membership fees. For many older adults and those with osteoporosis, walking has become a mainstay activity.

A walking program shouldn't be too easy or too hard. When you start, walk a short distance at a comfortable speed. Then gradually increase your distance but not the pace. As you feel yourself becoming better conditioned, you can begin a more formal program of fitness walking. This requires a speed of around 3 to 5 mph. A walking program should be done at least every other day to build both flexibility and endurance.

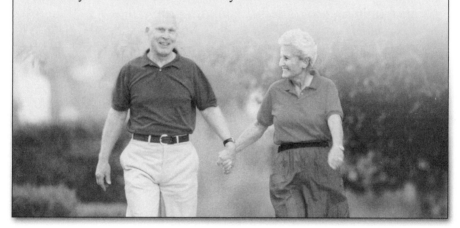

Resistance exercise

Whereas weight-bearing exercise uses gravity to strengthen the bones in your lower body, resistance exercise applies weight — or resistance — to specific muscles to strengthen them. Strong muscles allow you to stand up straight and move more assuredly, and they help keep you from falling. Activities that build muscle strength also work directly on bone to slow mineral loss.

To create resistance, your muscles have to push or pull against an opposing force. A common way to do resistance exercise is to lift weights, either with free weights or with weight machines. For this reason, resistance exercise is sometimes called weightlifting, weight training or strength training. But conditions such as osteoporosis make it difficult if not impossible to hoist heavy weights. Other, more gentle methods of resistance training include isometric exercises, resistance bands and water workouts.

Why do you need resistance exercise? As you grow older, your muscle fibers shrink in number and size. Sometime after age 30 your muscle mass begins to diminish by about 1 percent each year. That means you could be 40 percent weaker at age 70 than you were at 30. Losing muscle mass not only saps your strength but also affects your balance and coordination. Resistance exercise can slow or even reverse the age-related decline in muscle mass and bone density, help prevent compression fractures and stooped posture, and reduce the risk of falls.

If you have osteoporosis, you'll need assistance in designing a resistance-training program that includes proper lifting techniques and is appropriate for your degree of bone loss. Consult your doctor, a rehabilitation specialist (physiatrist), a registered physical therapist or a certified athletic trainer to determine what type of resistance exercise would be best for you.

Weight training. With proper supervision, many older adults, including those with osteoporosis, can participate in weightlifting. But you'll need to check with your doctor first. He or she can prescribe exercises based on your bone density and fitness level. The weights should be light. And you'll need to pay strict attention to proper technique to avoid placing too much stress on the spine.

Exercising with free weights is a great way to build muscle mass because it can simulate motions you make in real life, like carrying boxes or lifting a bag of groceries. Start with weights of 1 or 2 pounds — and not more than 5 pounds. You should be able to lift the weight comfortably at least eight times. One set of 10 lifts can effectively build muscle.

Free weights and weight machines can be found at most gyms and health clubs and in some schools. Often, instructors are available to assist you. You can make your own weights by filling old socks with beans or pennies or by partially filling a half-gallon jug with water or sand. Used weights also can be purchased by the pound at some athletic equipment stores. Often they'll be listed for sale in newspaper classified ads.

Isometric exercise. These exercises involve tensing your muscles while holding them in stationary positions. When you push your arm against a wall, for example, there's a buildup of tension in the muscles even though your arm isn't moving. Your own body creates the resistance.

Isometric exercises are especially useful for people recovering from injuries that limit range of motion. But don't do isometric exercises if you have high blood pressure or heart disease because your blood pressure can rise significantly during the muscle contractions.

Resistance bands. Large elastic or latex bands — they look just like large rubber bands — provide resistance when you pull on them. These exercise bands are made with different degrees of resistance to match your fitness level. Consult your doctor or an exercise specialist to select an appropriate resistance level. Someone with osteoporosis should start exercising with bands of low resistance. Resistance bands can easily be used at home or packed in a suitcase when you travel. Some bands have handles or an anchor so that they can be attached to a door.

Water workouts. Water offers resistance as you push against it. Simply walking in water with correct posture will strengthen your abdominal muscles. You can also perform upper and lower body moves such as squats and curls in the water. For a more intense workout, use barbells and weighted boots, which add to the water's natural resistance.

Many organizations, including YMCAs, YWCAs, health clubs and hospitals, offer water exercise classes. Look for an instructor who's certified in cardiopulmonary resuscitation (CPR) and trained in water safety instruction. Be sure to inform your instructor if you have a special condition such as osteoporosis or a heart condition that might affect your workout.

Several resistance exercises are shown on pages 134 and 135, but many others also may be suitable. Check with your doctor to make sure the exercises you choose are appropriate for you.

Move slowly and smoothly as you do these exercises. Inhale before you lift or exert, and exhale as you lift. Repeat each exercise 10 times, if possible.

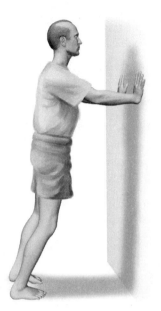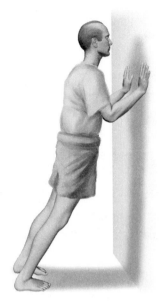

Wall push-ups. Face the wall, standing far enough away so that you can place your palms on the wall with your elbows slightly bent. Keeping your heels flat on the floor, slowly bend your elbows and lean toward the wall, supporting your weight with your arms. Try to keep your back straight. Straighten your arms and return to an upright position.

Chair sit-ups. Sit in a chair that has arms. Push your body up from the chair using your arms only. Hold this position for 10 seconds. Relax and repeat.

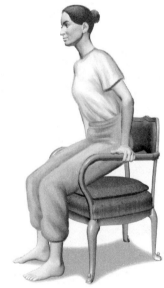

Stretching and flexibility

Stretching exercises help increase your flexibility, another key component of overall fitness. Flexibility is the capacity to move a body part, such as a leg or an arm, in different directions around a joint, such as a knee or an elbow. Having a maximum range of motion around a joint helps prevent muscle injury.

The specific exercises you perform may depend on your physical condition and exercise goals you've set for yourself. For example, for people with low bone density, the back-strengthening exercises described in this chapter may be useful.

Stretching exercises can be done every day, often in conjunction with weight-bearing exercise. The ideal time to stretch is when your muscles are loose — after you've exercised for 8 to 10 minutes. Forcing muscles to stretch without a warmup increases the risk of pulls.

Stretches should be gentle and slow. Stretch only until you feel a slight tension in the muscle. Relax and breathe deeply while you stretch. Hold your stretches for at least 30 seconds. It takes time to lengthen muscles safely.

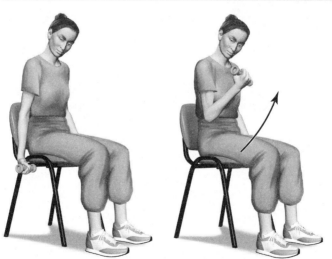

Biceps curls. Sitting in a chair, start with your arms at your sides. Bend one arm at the elbow, lifting a 1- or 2-pound weight to your shoulder without moving your shoulder or upper arm. Lower it slowly. Repeat with the other arm.

Back-strengthening exercise

Strengthening your back muscles may help treat osteoporosis by maintaining or improving posture. The stooped posture that results from compression fractures can increase the pressure along your spine, leading to more compression fractures. One way to prevent this from happening is to practice good posture.

Exercises that gently arch your back can strengthen back muscles and minimize stress on bones. Remember to avoid exercises that round your back because these activities can increase pressure on your spine.

A few back-strengthening exercises are described below, but you may also choose from many other exercises. Do this type of exercise once or twice a day. At the start, try to do at least three repetitions of each exercise, but don't do more than 10. Add new exercises or more repetitions only when the original set of exercises has become easy for at least 3 days. None of these exercises should hurt in any way while you're doing them or cause soreness for more than 1 day afterward.

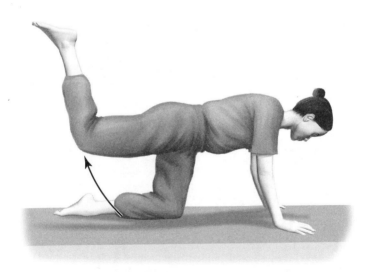

Lower back extensions. From a hands-and-knees position, raise one leg at the hip, keeping your knee bent and without changing the position of your trunk. Maintain this position for 5 seconds. Repeat exercise with the other leg.

Upper back extensions.
Sit forward on a chair, tuck
in your chin and relax your
shoulders. With elbows
bent and arms drawn back,
pull your shoulder blades
together as you straighten
your upper back. Inhale
deeply while gently pulling
your arms back. While
exhaling return to the starting position.

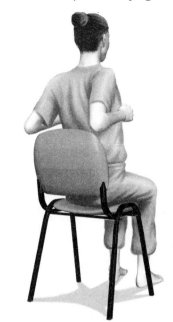

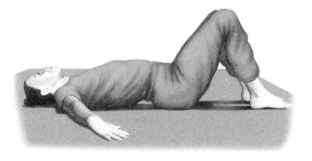

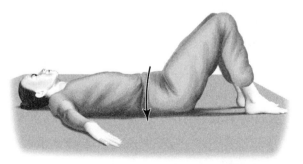

Pelvic tilts. Lie on the floor on your back with your knees bent
and feet resting flat on the floor. Tighten your abdominal muscles
as you roll your pelvis down, flattening the small of your back
against the surface. Avoid using your leg and buttock muscles.
Maintain this position for 5 seconds, then relax.

How much should you exercise?

Even if you've figured out which exercises you'll do, you may have other questions. How often should you exercise (frequency)? How hard a pace should you set (intensity)? How long should an exercise session last (duration)? Your doctor or physical therapist can help you answer all of these questions. Remember that it's best to start out at a comfortable level and, when you're ready, gradually increase your exertion. If you take more than a few days off, start back gradually, doing less than you were doing when you last exercised. Here are some other tips.

Frequency
To receive the maximum health benefits of exercise, try to do weight-bearing and back-strengthening exercises on most days of the week. Include resistance exercise two to three times a week.

Intensity
For weight-bearing exercise, start at a pace you can continue for 5 to 10 minutes without causing fatigue. As a rule of thumb, if you can't carry on a conversation while exercising, you're probably working too hard.

For most people, resistance exercise should be done at about 80 percent of their maximum muscle strength. Don't overexert yourself. This usually means lifting the same weight 8 to 10 times. In general, to promote bone strength, the intensity of your activities — how hard you work — should increase over time.

Duration
At the start, try to accumulate at least 30 minutes of weight-bearing exercise each day. This doesn't have to be accomplished all at one time. Rather, it's the total amount of activity you undertake in the course of a day, including routine tasks.

After a period of about 6 months — during which you've become fitter and gradually increased your activity — a daily exercise routine might include a 5-minute warm-up, 30 minutes of weight-bearing exercises and 5 to 10 minutes to cool down and stretch. Back-strengthening exercises may take 10 to 15 minutes. Two or three times a week include 10 to 20 minutes of resistance exercise. All of this activity can be broken into smaller sessions and spread throughout the day.

Staying in the game

For someone who is at risk of osteoporosis or already has it, activity and exercise plays an important part in preventing or managing the condition. No matter what exercise you undertake, the important thing is to get moving and make it a regular habit.

The key is attitude. If you can't seem to stick with an exercise program, you're probably missing a crucial ingredient — fun. If exercise is drudgery, you won't do it for long. Make exercise part of everyday activities and hobbies that you enjoy. Be active with friends and family members or choose an activity you've always wanted to try.

Here are other ways to stay motivated:
- If you're a beginner, set your sights on a 6-month exercise plan. People who stick with a new behavior for 6 months generally have long-term success — exercise becomes a habit.
- Choose exercises that fit your personality, physical health and lifestyle. Do you like to exercise alone or with a group? Do you like being outside or indoors?
- Join a class with people of a similar age and fitness level. Peer support can keep you going.
- Find an exercise buddy. Exercising with a companion is a great way to stay motivated. Encourage your friends and family to be active with you.
- Add variety to your exercise routine to prevent boredom. For example, alternate walking and bicycling with swimming or a low-impact aerobics class. On days when the weather is pleasant, do your back-strengthening exercises outside.
- Be flexible. If you're traveling or especially busy on a certain day, it's OK to adapt or shorten your exercise program to accommodate your schedule.

- Track your progress. Keeping a log helps you work toward your goals and reminds you of how far you've progressed.
- Reward yourself at milestones in your exercise plan. Schedule something special that you've always wanted to do. Attend a concert or social event, meet with a friend or go to your favorite restaurant.
- Forgive lapses. Everyone falls off the exercise wagon at some point. That's no excuse to quit. Remind yourself that it's just a temporary setback, and get moving again.

Being physically active on a regular basis is one of the most valuable gifts you can give yourself. Exercise can be as simple as a walk around the block or a few stretches while you listen to music. Being more active and eating a healthy diet are ways that you can take direct charge of your health and help manage conditions such as osteoporosis.

Chapter 10

Taking medications

Getting enough calcium and vitamin D in your diet and being physically active are key components of any action plan for osteoporosis. But these measures alone can't completely offset the bone loss due to aging and menopause in older adults. Similarly, these measures aren't sufficient to treat osteoporosis once you have the condition. So in addition to diet and exercise, medications are often prescribed to help slow bone loss and reduce your risk of fractures.

Your doctor may prescribe a medication to prevent or treat osteoporosis in these situations:

- You have low bone density, are postmenopausal or have other risk factors for osteoporosis.
- You've been diagnosed with osteoporosis.
- You experience continued bone loss or a fracture even though you have an adequate intake of calcium and vitamin D in your diet and are physically active.

In the past, the hormone estrogen was the treatment of choice for osteoporosis. Now a decision to use estrogen is more complex, given findings about the dangers of its long-term use from a recent study. Nevertheless, for short-term use, estrogen is effective and still prescribed for managing the changes of menopause, including age-related bone loss.

Other medications with fewer adverse effects than estrogen are effective options for the prevention and treatment of osteoporosis. These include a class of drugs known as bisphosphonates as well as raloxifene, calcitonin and a new drug derived from parathyroid hormone. The Food and Drug Administration (FDA) has approved all of these medications. Several medications now used for conditions other than osteoporosis, including zoledronic acid, pamidronate and thiazide diuretics, may also prove useful for strengthening bones. These medications are still under investigation and not approved by the FDA for treatment of osteoporosis.

Estrogen and hormone replacement therapy

For many years estrogen was considered the best way to prevent bone loss in women, although the effects of its long-term use were never studied. Estrogen was also prescribed to ease the symptoms of menopause, such as hot flashes, emotional upsets and mood swings, sleep disturbances, and vaginal and bladder changes.

Menopause generally occurs around the age of 50. During menopause a woman's ovaries produce significantly less estrogen and progesterone (pro-JES-tuh-rone), the two major female sex hormones. After menopause the production of the sex hormones drops to a fraction of what it used to be. Because of estrogen's key role in promoting bone health, during those first few years after menopause, bone density tends to decline at a rapid rate.

Hormone replacement therapy (HRT) supplements the natural estrogen that your body had produced in greater amounts before menopause. For women who haven't had a hysterectomy, a progestin (pro-JES-tin) is prescribed along with the estrogen. A progestin is one of several synthetic drugs that mimic the effects of progesterone. This combination is necessary because estrogen alone is known to increase the risk of uterine cancer in women. Progestin can protect the uterus from this problem. Women who have had a hysterectomy are able to take estrogen alone.

Hormone replacement therapy approximately doubles the amount of estrogen in your body after menopause. Even so, your estrogen level doesn't come close to pre-menopausal levels. Along with easing the symptoms of menopause, HRT effectively reduces bone breakdown and may result in a 5 percent to 6 percent increase in bone density of the lumbar vertebrae over 1 to 3 years of use. Studies show that HRT can also help prevent fractures of the hip, spine and other sites in your skeleton.

It has been estimated that in the mid-1990s, 35 percent to 40 percent of postmenopausal women in the United States used HRT. Many of these women discontinued HRT within 1 year for a variety of reasons. Others continued the treatment, sometimes into their 70s, because taking it made them feel better. Usage numbers for HRT have undergone a recent and dramatic reduction as new information about the effects of estrogen therapy emerges.

Risks of long-term use

Findings from the Women's Health Initiative (WHI), organized by the National Institutes of Health, have raised serious concerns about the long-term use of HRT. A WHI study was stopped prematurely in July 2002 because health risks for study participants being given Prempro, a combined estrogen and progestin pill, exceeded previously agreed upon limits for risk.

The study involved 16,000 women between ages 50 and 79. Approximately half of the participants were given Prempro and the other half given a placebo. The average amount of time that these women participated in the study was about 5 years. Increased risks for the women receiving Prempro included breast cancer, stroke, heart attack and serious blood clots (see sidebar "Women's Health Initiative results" on page 142). Study findings did, however, support the bone benefits of HRT over this time — the participants on Prempro had a risk reduction in total fractures and in hip fractures.

This WHI study didn't evaluate HRT taken in other doses or in the form of a patch, vaginal ring or cream — each of which may have its own set of risks and benefits. Also, the study found only modest benefits of estrogen for treating menopausal symptoms. Another WHI study evaluating the effect of taking estrogen alone, in pill form, is ongoing because risks have not exceeded the agreed-upon limits.

Women's Health Initiative results

In 2002 the National Institutes of Health ended one part of its Women's Health Initiative early because of serious health risks found among women in the study who were given hormone replacement therapy (HRT). In addition to risks, important benefits are associated with HRT, including fewer fractures.

Risks of taking Prempro
Annual occurrence per 10,000 women

	No Prempro	With Prempro
Breast cancer	30	38
Stroke	21	29
Heart attack	23	30
Serious blood clots	16	34

Benefits of taking Prempro
Annual occurrence per 10,000 women

	No Prempro	With Prempro
Colorectal cancer	16	10
Total fractures	19.1	14.7
Hip fractures	15	10

What are the implications?

Based on the WHI findings, 30 cases of invasive breast cancer would be expected every year from among 10,000 women who did not take Prempro. By comparison, 38 cases of invasive breast cancer would be expected from a population of the same size taking Prempro. The risks of stroke, heart attack and blood clots also showed a notable increase. These findings have provoked a dramatic re-evaluation of what had been a commonly accepted choice of treatment for many older women. At the same time, the numbers don't mean that you're destined to have breast cancer or a stroke just because you've taken or currently are taking HRT.

For women approaching menopause or going through menopause, the decision to take HRT has become that much more difficult. It's true that estrogen therapy is still the most effective course of treatment for hot flashes and other symptoms of menopause. Short-term use may be appropriate and seems to carry little risk. This therapy will protect your skeleton at the same time. Alternate treatments for menopausal symptoms include some lifestyle changes, dietary choices and nonhormonal prescription medications such as venlafaxine (Effexor) and gabapentin (Neurotin). Discuss the various options with your doctor.

What about using HRT to prevent or treat osteoporosis only? Long-term use (at least 5 years or more) carries the aforementioned risks from the WHI study. And research indicates that the beneficial effects of short-term therapy aren't permanent. Bone loss resumes as soon as HRT is discontinued. Currently, other medications are available that may be just as effective for your bone health but don't carry the risks of estrogen.

What if you've already been taking HRT for several years? You may be wondering when and how you should stop. Eventually, current and future studies will clarify the full effects of estrogen therapy on the human body, but until definitive answers are available, your treatment strategy should be the result of a careful and informed decision between you and your doctor. This decision can balance your health concerns with the known risks and benefits of HRT. Issues you'll likely consider include your personal and family history of diseases such as breast cancer or a history of blood clots, the reasons you're taking hormones, your health goals and the symptoms you're trying to eliminate. You might also consider other approaches that may prove as effective as estrogen.

If you choose to stop taking hormones, your doctor may recommend gradually reducing (tapering) the dosage of HRT over the course of several weeks to minimize the hot flashes that you may experience after you discontinue the medication. Because age-related bone loss resumes within 6 months of discontinuing HRT, it may be wise to start another form of osteoporosis prevention soon after. Talk to your doctor about other ways to manage your osteoporosis risk, such as diet and exercise and other medications.

Bisphosphonates

Bisphosphonates are antiresorptive (an-ih-ree-SORP-tiv) medications, meaning that they work by reducing bone resorption — the breakdown of bone tissue. The drugs alter the bone surface actions of the osteoclasts, the bone-excavating cells, and halt their functions. By doing so, bisphosphonates slow bone loss and increase the mineral content of bones, resulting in a stronger skeleton.

This class of medications includes alendronate (Fosamax) and risedronate (Actonel), both of which are commonly used in the United States. They generally increase bone density of the lumbar spine by 8 percent to 10 percent after 3 years of therapy, reduce the risk of new spinal fractures by 50 percent to 60 percent and reduce the risk of nonvertebral fractures by about 50 percent. These drugs are often prescribed for postmenopausal women, and they're often the first choice of treatment for men with osteoporosis. Alendronate and risedronate are also approved for the prevention and treatment of steroid-induced osteoporosis.

Although the long-term effectiveness and safety of these drugs haven't been studied, they have been used for over two decades without any apparent adverse effects. Your doctor may evaluate the safety and efficacy of your treatment on a yearly basis. Some experts recommend that bisphosphonates be used for about 4 years but there's good evidence that alendronate and risedronate are safe and effective for up to 7 years.

Other bisphosphonates being tested for possible long-term use include zoledronic acid (Zometa) and pamidronate (Aredia). Currently, both drugs are used to treat high levels of calcium in the bloodstream (hypercalcemia), which may occur with certain types of cancer. Although they aren't approved by the FDA for osteoporosis, they're sometimes used by people who can't tolerate the other bisphosphonates. The results of clinical trials are encouraging. A recent study of 351 postmenopausal women demonstrated that participants taking zoledronic acid in various dosages increased the bone density of the lumbar spine to 5 percent above that of women taking a placebo. Smaller studies have indicated that pamidronate is also effective.

Taking bisphosphonates. Alendronate and risedronate may be taken in pill form once a day or in a larger, once-a-week dose. Taking the medication once a week is just as effective as taking it daily and is more convenient for most people. A once-weekly dose may also result in fewer side effects.

These bisphosphonates are hard to digest for some people and can be hard on the digestive system. If taken with a meal, the drugs can bind to certain compounds in the food and leave the digestive tract without being absorbed. For this reason, bisphosphonates are taken on an empty stomach. To minimize any side effects, your doctor will recommend that you to take the pill first thing in the morning with a full glass (6 to 8 ounces) of water. After taking the pill, remain upright — sitting, standing or walking — for 30 minutes to ensure adequate absorption before eating, drinking anything other than plain water or ingesting other medications, including calcium supplements.

Zoledronic acid and pamidronate are administered with intravenous infusion once a year. Because these medications enter the bloodstream directly via injection, only small doses of it are needed to slow bone breakdown. These drugs effectively stop bone loss for up to 12 months after they're given.

Side effects. The side effects of bisphosphonates are generally mild. Taking alendronate or risedronate may produce gastrointestinal problems such as heartburn, indigestion, nausea, diarrhea and pain when swallowing. These effects may be reduced by carefully following the instructions for taking the medication. The side effects of zoledronic acid include body aches, low-grade fever, bone pain and eye inflammation.

Teriparatide

Parathyroid hormone (PTH) is produced by the parathyroid glands, which are located behind the thyroid gland at the base of your neck. PTH plays a critical role in the bone remodeling cycle and in maintaining the calcium balance in your bloodstream. This hormone can raise the calcium level in your blood by several means. It increases how much calcium is absorbed in your intestines, releases stored calcium in your bones and reduces the amount of calcium excreted by your kidneys. Although large amounts of PTH can cause bone loss, small doses of the hormone can strengthen bones.

Teriparatide (Forteo) is derived from PTH. It's called an anabolic agent because it builds new bone. It works by stimulating the osteoblast cells and, by so doing, increases bone building. All other medications currently approved for treating osteoporosis are antiresorptives, which work by decreasing bone breakdown.

Researchers studying 1,637 postmenopausal women who had osteoporosis and a history of spinal fractures found that daily injections of teriparatide, along with calcium and vitamin D supplementation, increased bone density of the spine by 9 percent to 13 percent over the control group taking a placebo with supplementation. The medication also reduced the risk of fractures in other bones by 35 percent to 54 percent.

A warning that accompanies the drug notifies you of studies on laboratory rats that developed malignant bone tumors after being given doses of teriparatide far greater than the dosage given to humans. The FDA continues to monitor these tests. In spite of this warning, teriparatide appears to be safe and the chance of a similar outcome occurring in humans seems unlikely.

Teriparatide is taken by daily, self-administered injections in your thigh or abdomen. Your supply comes in a disposable device that looks like a fat ballpoint pen. The device contains 28 doses — enough to last 1 month — before it needs to be replaced. Teriparatide may be used to treat women and men with severe forms of osteoporosis, including those who are at high risk of fractures or who haven't responded well to other forms of treatment, such as antiresorptive drugs.

The optimal length of treatment with teriparatide hasn't been established. Because the long-term effectiveness and safety of the medication aren't known, the FDA advises that treatment should continue for no longer than 2 years. Teriparatide is very expensive compared with other medications for treating osteoporosis. At the end of treatment with this anabolic agent, an antiresorptive drug may be prescribed to maintain the gains in bone mass.

Raloxifene

Raloxifene (Evista) belongs to a class of drugs called selective estrogen receptor modulators (SERMs). SERMs are sometimes referred to as designer estrogens because their chemical structure has been manipulated, or designed, in a laboratory. These synthetic compounds mimic some of estrogen's beneficial effects while avoiding some, but not all, of its adverse effects.

SERMs work by either activating or inhibiting estrogen receptors in tissue that have these receptors, such as bones and breast tissue. This means that sometimes the drugs act just like estrogen, and at other times they block the effects of estrogen. For example, raloxifene binds to estrogen receptors in bone cells, which may then cause an increase in bone density in much the same way estrogen does. But when raloxifene interacts with estrogen receptors in breast tissue, the drug blocks the action of estrogen. This may lessen your breast cancer risk, as suggested by findings from a study testing the effects of raloxifene on bone.

Raloxifene slows bone loss to a degree similar to that of estrogen. Among postmenopausal women with osteoporosis who were studied for 3 years, daily treatment with raloxifene reduced the risk of vertebral fractures by 36 percent. However, treatment has not proven to significantly reduce other types of fractures, such as the wrist or hip. Other studies have shown that raloxifene produces small increases in bone mass of the spine, hip and total body.

Raloxifene was initially developed as a treatment for breast cancer and is similar to tamoxifen, another SERM. When researchers discovered that raloxifene had a positive effect on bone density, their focus shifted to its use as a treatment for osteoporosis. Raloxifene appears to have the additional benefit of reducing the risk of breast cancer without increasing the risk of uterine cancer.

Taking raloxifene. Raloxifene is available as a 60-milligram tablet. You take one tablet each day, preferably at the same time of day. It can be taken with or without food.

Side effects. Leg cramps and hot flashes are the most commonly reported side effects. Other possible problems include leg swelling and an influenza-like syndrome.

Like estrogen, raloxifene increases the risk of blood clots by approximately threefold, but the risk that an individual woman will have this problem is very low. For example, among approximately 155 women treated with raloxifene for 3 years, one blood clot would be diagnosed. Nevertheless, your doctor may recommend that you avoid this medication if you have a history of blood clots or are at risk of developing them.

Calcitonin

Calcitonin is a hormone produced in the thyroid gland. It may help regulate the amount of calcium circulating in the bloodstream. During pregnancy and breast-feeding, the amount of calcitonin released by the thyroid increases considerably, which may help to protect a woman's skeleton as her need for calcium increases.

A synthetic form of calcitonin is approved by the FDA to treat, but not prevent, postmenopausal osteoporosis. Like the bisphosphonates and raloxifene, calcitonin is an antiresorptive drug, which works by slowing bone breakdown. Calcitonin comes in two forms, an injectable version (Calcimar, Cibacalcin) and a nasal spray (Miacalcin). The nasal spray is the most commonly used form.

Calcitonin is safer but less effective than other medications for osteoporosis. For that reason, it's often considered one of the last treatment options after bisphosphonates, teriparatide and raloxifene. Calcitonin may slow bone loss and increase bone density modestly, and it has been found to reduce the risk of vertebral fractures by 36 percent. The drug hasn't been found to decrease a person's risk of hip fracture. Calcitonin may also relieve bone pain in people with osteoporotic spinal fractures, especially in the first weeks after a fracture.

Calcitonin is generally used to treat women who are at high risk of fracture and can't take bisphosphonates or raloxifene. It's also used to treat men who can't tolerate the bisphosphonates.

Taking calcitonin. The injectable form of calcitonin must be taken daily. The method is similar to injecting insulin for diabetes. Your doctor can help you learn the proper technique for adminis-

Medications for men with osteoporosis

To date, only two medications — alendronate (Fosamax) and parathyroid hormone (Forteo) — have been approved by the Food and Drug Administration (FDA) for the treatment of osteoporosis in men. Along with alendronate, risedronate (Actonel) is approved for treating osteoporosis that occurs in men and women as a result of long-term use of steroids such as prednisone or cortisone.

To help men with osteoporosis, doctors may also prescribe the following:

- **Testosterone.** Testosterone replacement therapy is used only for men who have osteoporosis caused by low testosterone levels. Taking it when you have normal testosterone levels won't increase bone density.
- **Calcitonin.** This medication slows or stops bone loss and may relieve the pain of spinal fractures. It's sometimes used to treat men (and women) who are at high risk of fractures but who can't tolerate bisphosphonates such as alendronate. The effects of calcitonin in men haven't been studied, but evidence suggests that it may work the same in men as it does in women.

Certain drugs used to treat osteoporosis in women should not be used in men:

- **Estrogen.** In men this hormone can cause blood clots, breast enlargement and lowered sex drive.
- **Raloxifene (Evista).** This drug is approved only for women with osteoporosis. More research is needed before this estrogen-like drug is used in men.

All men need to take care that they get enough calcium and vitamin D. Men under age 65 need about 1,000 mg of calcium each day, and men age 65 and older should consume at least 1,500 mg. See "Assessing your calcium intake" in Chapter 8 to learn how much you may currently consume in your diet.

tering this injection. The nasal spray is taken by spraying one puff in one nostril each day, alternating nostrils. You can take calcitonin with or without food.

Refrigerate the nasal spray medication until opened, then keep it at room temperature and covered.

Side effects. With the injectable form of calcitonin, side effects are more common and more bothersome, occurring in about 20 percent of people who use this form of the drug. Side effects include nausea, vomiting, irritation at the injection site and flushing of the face and hands.

The only serious side effect of the nasal spray is nasal irritation or discomfort, which occurs in about 12 percent of people taking the drug.

Medications under investigation

Research is ongoing for several experimental treatments that may prevent bone breakdown or stimulate the formation of new bone. Investigators are looking for medications that are effective, easy to take, inexpensive and have few side effects.

Thiazide diuretics

Thiazide diuretics are used primarily to lower blood pressure by reducing the volume of water in the body. But several studies have shown that thiazide diuretics can also increase bone density. This may occur because diuretics reduce the amount of calcium that the kidneys excrete into urine. Because less calcium passes out of the body, more may be available for storage in your bones.

Thiazides may be useful in preventing osteoporosis, but they're not used solely for that purpose. For people with high blood pressure, thiazides may be a good choice of treatment because they can help preserve bone density as they lower blood pressure.

Sodium fluoride

Sodium fluoride is commonly used on children's teeth to help prevent cavities. For years the mineral has been used experimentally to treat osteoporosis. Sodium fluoride is known to stimulate bone formation and increase bone density. However, the new bone that is formed is abnormal and less flexible than normal bone. And fluoride hasn't been shown to reduce the risk of fractures — it may even increase the risk of hip fractures. Currently, fluoride isn't recommended for treating osteoporosis, although slow-release forms of fluoride are being studied to see if they may be more effective with fewer of the risks to your skeleton.

Vitamin D analogues

Vitamin D undergoes several conversions as it's processed in the body. Each conversion produces a new compound that is essential for the next conversion to take place. These various forms (analogues) of vitamin D are being studied as possible treatments for osteoporosis. Alfacalcidol (One-Alpha) and calcitriol (Calcijex, Rocaltrol) are vitamin D compounds used in other countries to treat osteoporosis. These medications increase bone density in the spine, but their effect on fractures is unknown.

Growth hormone and growth factors

Growth hormone (somatotropin) is produced by the pituitary gland in your brain. The hormone plays a major role in stimulating bone growth during childhood and adolescence. It also affects bone remodeling in adults, but whether growth hormone can be used to prevent or treat bone loss is unclear.

Growth factors are proteins that promote skeletal growth, help repair body tissues and stimulate the production of blood cells. Laboratory studies indicate that they build bone, but they still haven't been tested in clinical trials.

Ipriflavone

Ipriflavone is a synthetic compound that belongs to a class of substances called isoflavones, a type of phytoestrogen. Phytoestrogens are estrogens that occur in plant foods such as soybeans. Although preliminary research indicates that ipriflavone may prevent bone loss, its effect is modest, and the drug doesn't seem to prevent fractures in women with osteoporosis.

Evaluating your options

In the last two decades, new medications for osteoporosis have helped to transform what was an insidious and unpredictable disorder into a treatable condition, similar to the effect that new medications have had on high blood pressure. The new medications hold promise not only in stopping the breakdown of bone but also in promoting bone growth, turning net bone loss into bone gain. You and your doctor now have a variety of options from which to choose the most effective drug to fit your individual needs.

Whatever your course of treatment, to receive the full benefit of your action plan, it's essential that you take these medications as prescribed by your doctor. It's also important to stay active and to maintain an adequate intake of calcium and vitamin D in your diet. This will maximize the effectiveness of your medications.

Chapter 11

Living with osteoporosis

O steoporosis may be thought of as a bone disease, but its impact extends well beyond your skeleton. Many people with osteoporosis learn to live with the condition as they go about their daily activities. But for others, especially those who have fractured a bone, osteoporosis can take a tremendous physical, emotional and social toll.

If you have osteoporosis, work and household tasks may become more difficult and require others' assistance. You may be subject to chronic pain and fatigue. You may experience stress, anxiety, fear, isolation, depression and loss of self-esteem. Your social relationships may be harder to maintain. You may not be as independent and active as you once were.

Coping with any chronic illness requires patience, perseverance and self-acceptance. You don't have to give in to despair or avoid your normal routines. You can maintain your quality of life even if you have fractures or pain due to osteoporosis.

This chapter presents strategies to help you cope with some of the physical, emotional and social aspects of having osteoporosis. Coping may require a team effort involving family and friends, your doctor and other health professionals. Above all, it requires your commitment to improving your health and keeping your outlook positive.

Practice good posture

If you're living with osteoporosis, you're living with greater risk of injury from movements that involve twisting, lifting, carrying or bending. But being cautious doesn't mean you stop being active.

You can take steps to increase your safety and protect yourself from fractures and falls. Learning to sit, stand and move using good posture and body mechanics makes it easier to function in your daily routine. Poor posture increases the strain on your muscles and bones, causes fatigue and makes you more prone to injury. Ingrained habits of poor posture can complicate a condition such as osteoporosis. Throughout the day, including when you exercise, try to maintain good posture. By making sure you're moving safely, you can accomplish many of the tasks you set out to do.

Straighten up

Start by knowing what *not* to do. If you have osteoporosis, even mild strains and pressure can cause a fracture. It's important to avoid bending forward, especially during activities that involve lifting or reaching. Also avoid excessive twisting of the spine. Here are some tips that can help you improve your posture:

- Think tall when you stand. Keep your stomach muscles tight.
- Stand with your weight on both feet.
- Wear comfortable shoes without high heels.
- When standing in one place, put one foot up on a stool or chair rung and switch to the other foot periodically.
- Don't carry a shoulder bag that weighs more than 2 pounds.
- Sit in a straight-back chair with your back supported.
- When you're seated, the chair seat should be high enough that your thighs rest horizontally on the seat and your feet are flat on the floor.
- When sitting for long periods, occasionally elevate your legs by placing your feet on a footstool. Also change positions to shift your weight. If possible, get up and move around every half-hour or so.
- When seated in bucket seats or soft chairs, use a thick rolled-up towel or pillow to support your lower back.

Are you standing tall?

One way to correct your standing posture is with the wall test. Stand with the back of your head, shoulder blades and buttocks against a wall and your heels 2 to 4 inches from the wall.

Check the curve of your lower spine by placing your flattened hand behind the small of your back. You should be able to fit your hand snugly between your lower back and the wall. If you can fit more than a hand's thickness between your lower back and the wall, adjust your pelvis to decrease the space.

If you have difficulty placing your hand between your lower back and the wall, increase the space to attain a good posture.

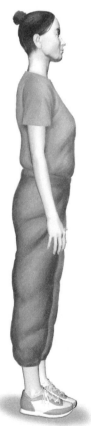

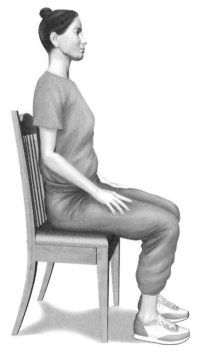

Good sitting posture: Spine and head erect, back and legs at a 90-degree angle, natural curves of the back are maintained.

Good standing posture: Head erect with chin tucked in, chest held high, shoulders relaxed, hips level, knees straight but not locked, feet parallel.

Coughing and sneezing

The force of a cough or sneeze can cause you to jerk forward suddenly, which may result in a compression fracture. To avoid such injury, develop the habit of placing your hand behind your back or on your thigh for support.

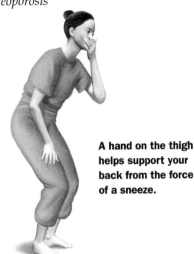

A hand on the thigh helps support your back from the force of a sneeze.

Sleeping positions

Avoid aggravating your back and maintain your spine's normal curve when you sleep or lie down.

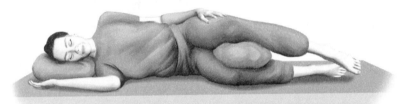

Sleep on your side with your thighs somewhat drawn up toward your chest. Place a pillow between your legs.

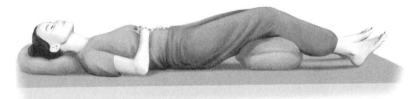

If you sleep on your back, support your knees and neck with pillows.

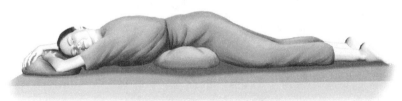

Sleep on your stomach only if a pillow cushions your abdomen.

Use proper movements

Always strive to use good posture and body mechanics as you go about your daily activities. Look for new and more efficient ways to perform them. You don't necessarily have to do things because "That's the way I've always done them." Avoid movements such as reaching, bending, twisting or using short, choppy motions, which can be dangerous for someone with osteoporosis. Here are tips for performing common tasks in a safe manner:

Lifting. Lifting objects, even objects that are lightweight, puts stress on your spine. To lift properly, keep your feet about shoulder-width apart and maintain the normal curve of your spine. Place one foot forward, and lower your body down to one knee by bending at the hips and knees, keeping your body weight on the balls of your feet.

- Make sure that you're close to the object you're about to lift. If the object is heavy, lift it first to your bent knee.
- Grasping the object, rise from the floor by using your leg muscles. Gently breathe in while you're straightening up. Don't hold your breath.
- Carry the object close to your body at about waist level. If possible, place your forearms under the object. Turn by pivoting your feet. Don't twist at your waist.

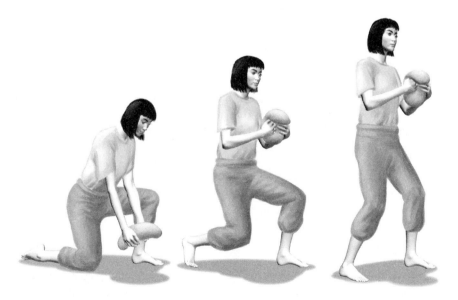

Pushing and pulling. To move objects, try to minimize the strain put on your back. If possible, push rather than pull.

- Bend your knees so that your arms are level with the object. Don't bend forward at the waist.
- Maintain the normal curve of your spine and walk forward or backward, using your body weight to push or pull the object.

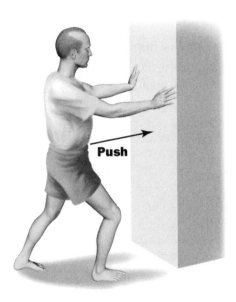

Push

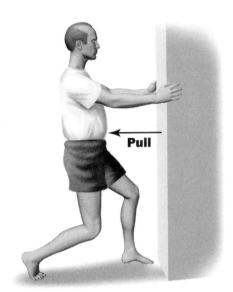

Pull

Using long-handled tools. The movements of sweeping, vacuuming and raking can put undue stress on your spine.

- Stand with one foot forward. Use a rocking motion to shift your body weight to your forward foot. To pull back, shift your weight to your back foot.
- Use arm and leg movements instead of back movements.
- Avoid overreaching, twisting and choppy motions. Use long, smooth strokes.

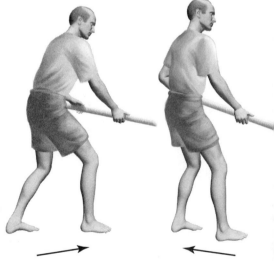

Safety tips for common daily tasks

- If you're sweeping, use a long-handled dustpan.
- Use casters under your furniture to make moving it easier.
- An upright vacuum requires you to stoop less. Self-propelled vacuums also are easier to use.
- For mopping, fill the pail half full and lower it to the floor using both hands. Finish filling the pail with a smaller container. After mopping, empty the pail halfway using the container, then lift the bucket and dump it into the sink.
- When changing bedding, avoid using fitted sheets unless you have a single bed or a lightweight mattress. You can tuck in the corners of a flat sheet using an open hand. If you must lift the mattress, get help.
- Carry a laundry basket that's only half full or use a basket on wheels. Be sure you can see the floor when you're walking with the basket, especially when you're on the stairs.
- Use an ironing board that's at the correct height for you. Have a clothes rack nearby to hang your ironed clothes on. And when you sort clothing, do so at a table or counter that doesn't require you to hunch forward while working.
- Drive up to the parcel pickup for your groceries or have your groceries delivered. Never attempt to carry them yourself, even if they seem lightweight.

Boost your emotional health

Having osteoporosis may stir a wide range of emotions. And the more severe your condition, the more intense your emotions are likely to be. When you first learn you have the disease, you may feel shock, disbelief or anger. If you've fractured a bone, you may feel helpless. Anxiety and depression also are common responses.

Negative emotions are a natural and understandable reaction to a chronic illness. Such emotions don't have to get the best of you. For many people the first step is admitting that their negative feelings exist. This can be tough in a culture that so frequently praises the optimist and criticizes the complainer.

Fear and anxiety

"What happens if I fracture a bone?" This is one of the most common fears among people with osteoporosis. You may worry that a fracture will result in the loss of your independence and require you to depend on others. You may feel anxious if you can't live up to your own or others' expectations, for example, if your condition limits your ability to cook, clean or care for yourself.

Fear of fracture often leads a person to limit his or her activities. This can set off a vicious cycle: A more sedentary lifestyle leads to decreased physical conditioning, making you more susceptible to falls, which in turn makes you all the more reluctant to be active. Lack of activity can also lead to apathy, isolation and depression.

Depression

Studies indicate that up to 50 percent of people with a chronic illness will also have depression. Having osteoporosis, you're most likely to develop depression if you're no longer able to carry out daily tasks or if you're experiencing pain from fractures. Anxiety, reduced activity and changes in your physical appearance also may contribute to depression.

Depression can manifest itself in a variety of ways that you may not always recognize:

- Sleep problems
- Changes in appetite
- Loss of interest or pleasure in most activities
- Irritability and mood swings
- Restlessness
- Feelings of hopelessness, worthlessness or guilt
- Extreme fatigue or loss of energy
- Decreased concentration, attention and memory

If you think you might be depressed, talk to your doctor, a mental health professional such as a psychiatrist or psychologist, or a social worker. It's important to get treatment because untreated depression can raise your risk of other health problems. With treatment, most people who have depression show improvement, often in a matter of weeks. Treatment may include medication, psychotherapy or both.

Anger

It's natural to become angry when you're confronting a chronic illness, pain or disability. But it's unhealthy to stay angry, bottle up your feelings or express them through explosive outbursts.

Mismanaged anger, whether it's short term and intense or lingering and subdued, can lead to headaches, backaches, high blood pressure and other health problems. Anger also increases muscle tension, making it difficult to relax. Your goal is not to abolish anger but to find healthier ways of dealing with the emotion.

Controlling stress

No one is immune from stress, but a chronic condition such as osteoporosis can ratchet up your stress level. Sometimes simply becoming aware of the causes can make stress easier to deal with. Aim for a healthy balance of activities in your day — time for work, physical activity, socializing, relaxation and rest. These stress-relieving tactics may help:

Plan your day. A plan can help you feel more in control of your life. You might start by getting out of bed 15 minutes earlier to ease the morning rush. Keep a written schedule of your daily activities so that you don't run into conflicts or last-minute panics to get to an appointment.

Plan before you act. Before you begin a task, gather all of the items you need. For example, keep cleaning supplies in one bucket to avoid multiple trips up and down the stairs. Or list the items you need before shopping, to avoid a second trip.

Keep commonly used items accessible. Organize your living space and work space so that the items you use frequently are close at hand. For example, keep your wrenches and screwdrivers on a pegboard above the workbench. Keep frequently used files on your desk.

Break apart lengthy tasks. Avoid spending too much time on one activity. Instead of spending all day planting your garden, spend 1 or 2 hours a day in the garden over 3 or 4 days.

Work at a moderate pace. Instead of rushing to complete a task, take your time and work at a comfortable speed.

Issues of self-esteem

Osteoporosis can deliver a blow to your self-esteem. If multiple fractures prevent you from working at a job, pursuing a hobby or doing household chores, you might feel less competent. Feelings of worthlessness can send your self-esteem spiraling downward.

Your self-image may suffer from physical changes, such as stooped posture brought on by compression fractures of your vertebrae. You may lose height and weight, or your abdomen may protrude. You may see yourself as somehow deformed.

The physical changes that occur with osteoporosis can be especially challenging in a society that so highly values youthful beauty and vigor. Under normal circumstances, these ideals are hard enough to fulfill. With fractures from osteoporosis, meeting expectations becomes even more elusive.

Coping strategies

The following strategies can help you reduce stress, anxiety and depression and boost your self-esteem. Research shows that people diagnosed with osteoporosis can improve their emotional well-being by being actively involved in their health management.

Educate yourself. The more you know about osteoporosis, the less abstract and threatening it will seem. Fear of the unknown can cause anxiety. Understanding can calm fear. If you're afraid of falling, for example, you can minimize the risks by learning how to move safely. You'll also know that doing no activity only makes you less fit and more prone to falls.

Exercise. Research shows that regular exercise reduces the symptoms of anxiety and plays a role in treating mild to moderate depression. Exercise also promotes a better self-image and raises self-esteem. For more information about physical activity and osteoporosis, see Chapter 9.

Learn to relax. Relaxation helps to counteract stress. Relaxation can also help you cope with daily demands and remain energetic and productive. Many techniques promote relaxation, including deep breathing, progressive muscle relaxation, meditation, biofeedback, hypnosis and guided imagery. It may be helpful to learn about the various relaxation techniques from a physical therapist.

Looking good

Feeling good about how you look is closely tied to self-esteem. But finding nice-looking clothes that fit well can be challenging for some people with osteoporosis. Compression fractures of your vertebrae may cause you to lose height and develop a curved back or a protruding abdomen. Blouses and shirts may feel too tight, skirts and pants may ride too high, and dresses may appear too short in the back and too long in the front.

If you can sew, try modifying clothing patterns or tailoring store-bought clothes. Otherwise, consider the following tips when buying clothing:

- Look for blouses or shirts with loosefitting sleeves, for example, dolman or raglan sleeves. Also try blouses with shoulder pads.
- Choose straight-sided jackets, blazers, shirts and dresses. Go for a boxy, unstructured look. Avoid clothes that accentuate the waistline.
- Buy clothes a size larger than you usually buy. A snug fit can draw attention to bumps and bulges you may wish unnoticed.
- Use accessories such as scarves or hats to jazz up a simple ensemble.
- To minimize the abdomen, women can wear dresses with dropped waistlines.
- Women can experiment with different types of bras, such as front-closure bras, sports bras or those with crisscross straps, to find one that fits well and is comfortable.

Adapted from the National Osteoporosis Foundation, 2000

Practice positive thinking. A coping technique that many people find effective is positive self-talk. Self-talk is the endless stream of thoughts that run through your head every day. These thoughts may be positive or negative.

With practice you can learn to recognize negative thoughts and replace them with positive ones. For example, if your negative thought is, "I can't do things the way I used to — I'm useless," you can replace it with a positive thought such as, "I can do much of what I want to do. As long as I don't overdo it, I can still be active." Over time, positive self-talk will become more automatic.

Manage your anger. Learn to identify what triggers your anger and recognize the warning signs. When you find yourself becoming angry, take a short timeout. Remember that you have a choice in how to respond to situations. Look for ways to release strong emotions, such as writing, listening to music, gardening or painting.

Many of these coping strategies will have a positive effect on your self-esteem. Here are some other ideas for building a strong sense of self-worth:

- Structure your day with goals you can achieve. When the day is done, you'll feel a sense of accomplishment.
- Seek emotional support. Reach out to family and friends. Confer with a counselor or a mental health professional.
- Help someone else. It reminds you that your life makes a difference.
- Treat yourself to something you enjoy, such as music, a book, a movie or going out with a friend.

Maintain social connections

For many people a satisfying social life is the key to feeling good mentally and physically. Social ties can give you a sense of purpose in life. And staying connected is good for your health. Studies show that people with strong social support recover from illness better than do people who face illness alone. A network of family and friends helps you to recover from any injury, including a fracture. Social contact can motivate you to be more involved in living.

Social consequences of osteoporosis
Osteoporosis can affect your relationships with family and friends in a number of ways. Most of us define ourselves to some extent by the social positions we hold, such as parent, spouse, colleague or manager. Even mild osteoporosis can change these relationships.

You may become more dependent on your spouse or adult children. You may lose a sense of shared effort and contribution within the family or at work. You may not be able to reciprocate friends' good will and intentions. Depending on the severity of your condition or your risk of fracture, you may have to let go of some or all of your job and household responsibilities.

People with severe osteoporosis may withdraw socially because of chronic pain or fear of fractures. If you suffer from chronic pain, riding in a car, sitting in a hard chair, standing or walking can quickly become uncomfortable. To avoid the pain, you may start avoiding some of your customary activities, such as attending religious services, playing cards, going to movies and traveling.

Fear of falling down also can result in social isolation. You may avoid going out in public, especially to crowded places, because you worry about being pushed or stumbling. You may no longer shop at grocery stores or malls because lifting and carrying bags can be difficult.

Reach out to family and friends

Many of us are used to being quite independent — and we're happy that way. It may seem embarrassing to ask others for help, especially with tasks you've done all of your life. But this is a time to put your safety and personal needs above your autonomy.

Although relying on others might seem unnatural at first, this increased reliance can actually help you manage your physical health and stay independent. For example, by asking someone to help you with day-to-day tasks such as shopping and housework that requires lifting, you reduce the risk of fracture. It's not a sign of weakness to ask for assistance when you need it.

It's true that relationships can sometimes be as much a source of stress as support. Your loved ones may not understand everything you're going through emotionally, but they're most likely eager to help you adjust. They can provide encouragement, offer gentle but helpful feedback and lend a hand when you need it. Good relationships require patience, compromise and acceptance. Your family and friends will need to accept your needs just as you must learn to accept theirs.

Bolster your social network

Does your social network need a boost? Consider these tips:

- Make it a point to answer all phone calls, e-mail and letters from family and friends.
- Accept invitations to social events.
- Take the initiative and invite someone to join in an activity.
- Become more involved in community organizations, neighborhood events and family get-togethers.
- At local gatherings, strike up a conversation when the opportunity arises.
- Join a group exercise class that's safe for someone with osteoporosis. Your doctor can advise what's appropriate.
- Set aside any past differences with friends and approach each relationship with a clean slate.

Join a support group

It's discouraging to feel that no one else understands exactly what you're going through. In fact, there *are* people who understand, primarily because they're going through it themselves. Support groups, also called self-help groups, bring together people who share common concerns. Even if your family is sympathetic, sometimes it's helpful to talk with others in a similar situation.

A support group can give you a sense of belonging. It gives you a place to express your feelings and fears and to exchange experiences. It also provides an opportunity to meet new friends.

Support groups may vary in format and size, but they're all based on peer support. Meetings are usually held in a library, hospital or community center. Many groups are sponsored by a hospital or a clinic or led by a health professional. The National Osteoporosis Foundation has developed a national network of affiliated support groups called Building Strength Together. To find an osteoporosis support group in your area, ask your doctor or contact the National Osteoporosis Foundation at *www.nof.org* or (800) 223-9994.

Chapter 12

Recovering from a fracture

You didn't plan on spending the next 4 to 8 months recovering from hip surgery. Then again, you didn't plan on slipping in the bathtub and breaking your hip either. And now here you are, using a walker to move around the house. You need help doing tasks like the laundry and making dinner. You can't get out to see friends like you used to. You feel like you'll never be your old self again.

It's true that recuperating from a broken bone, particularly an osteoporotic fracture, can be painful, time-consuming and frustrating. But many people do regain their former abilities and a semblance of their former life. In general, the healthier you are and the more positive your attitude, the better equipped you are for recovery from a fracture.

In this chapter you'll learn how bone naturally heals and restores itself after breaking. The discussion also includes forms of treatment for the most common osteoporotic fractures — those of the spine, hip and wrist — and what's involved in each rehabilitation phase. The chapter also examines various ways to manage chronic pain, which is sometimes a residual effect of osteoporotic fracture. Learning about the type of fracture you may have and the treatment that's available can help hasten your recovery and get you active again.

The nature of your recovery

How well you recover from a broken bone depends in part on the location and severity of the fracture. In many instances, prompt medical attention and the body's natural healing process lead to fracture repair within several months. For example, a wrist fracture will usually heal if you wear a cast and arm sling until your wrist is stable enough to bear weight again.

But it's not always that straightforward. Additional support may be needed for severe breaks, such as hip fractures, which generally require surgery. Other fractures, such as vertebral fractures, often cause chronic pain after the bone is healed and require a different therapeutic approach.

You'll find that each fracture has its own course of treatment. In addition to healing the bone, you may also receive treatment for osteoporosis, if you haven't started already, to increase your bone density.

But the recovery process doesn't necessarily end once the bone is healed. You may wish to reclaim most, if not all, of the life you led before you broke the bone. Ongoing therapy may return most of your former strength and mobility. You can use various techniques and devices to compensate for any permanent loss. In addition, you can work to prevent other fractures. This often involves using diet, exercise, medications and some lifestyle changes to maintain bone density.

How bone heals

As described in Chapter 2, your bones are continuously renewing themselves in a process called the remodeling cycle. Cells called osteoclasts tear down, or resorb, old or damaged bone while cells called osteoblasts build new bone. The remodeling cycle is the basis of fracture healing. In fact, bone is the only solid tissue in your body that can replace itself. Other tissue injuries, such as a skin wound, heal with the formation of a different, fibrous tissue that leaves a scar.

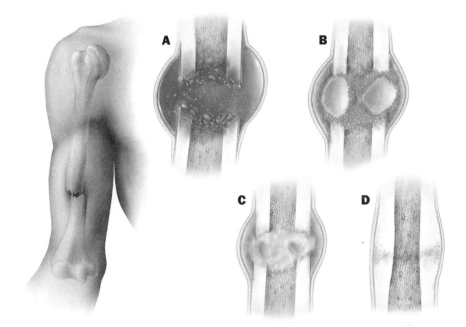

How a broken bone heals

After a break, a blood clot forms, sealing off damaged blood vessels between the ends of the broken bones (A). A soft callous develops as the bone begins to regenerate (B). Osteoblasts help to build a mesh of spongy bone, creating an internal splint that links the fractured bone ends (C). With the deposit of calcium and other minerals, this mesh develops into denser bone (D).

Self-repair of a bone fracture can be described in phases:

Phase 1. When a bone breaks, it bleeds just like any other tissue in the body. A blood clot forms that seals off damaged blood vessels in or near the broken bone. Scientists believe that molecules in the blood clot signal specialized cells to help with the repair process, such as immune cells that fight infection and growth factor cells that regulate tissue growth. Meanwhile, osteoclasts begin removing damaged bone and tissue. The initial phase generally takes about 2 weeks.

Phase 2. Over the next 4 weeks, the bone begins to regenerate with the help of osteoblasts. A soft callous forms made of collagen, the structural framework of bone.

Phase 3. The work of the osteoblasts continues as a mesh of spongy bone develops. This creates an internal splint linking the fractured bone ends.

Phase 4. Within 6 to 12 weeks of the fracture, denser, harder bone replaces the mesh of spongy bone. Newly deposited minerals in the collagen bind together and harden, resulting in greater bone strength. At this point, the fracture may be considered healed, although remodeling continues modify and strengthen the bone for at least a year or two.

Throughout this process, the fractured bone must be correctly aligned to allow proper healing. Problems usually arise when the ends of the fractured bone aren't aligned or can't be immobilized. In such instances, surgery or other medical procedures may be necessary to reposition the bones and stabilize the fracture.

Treating vertebral fractures

When bone density decreases due to osteoporosis, the vertebrae in your spinal column start to weaken. Eventually, some vertebrae lose most of their mineral content. The impact from falling down or the twisting of your torso can cause a compression fracture. So can lifting a load that is too heavy for your vertebrae to bear. The vertebral body literally collapses and falls in on itself. Although some compression fractures produce no symptoms, others can cause a sudden, sharp pain or pain that is chronic and persistent.

Generally, fractures of the vertebrae can be treated with pain relievers, bed rest, braces worn around the midsection and physical therapy. Compression fractures usually heal within 2 to 4 months, and acute pain gradually recedes during this period. Sometimes the pain may persist and isn't relieved by these conventional methods. In these instances, surgical procedures may be considered for treatment of fractures that cause chronic, unrelieved pain.

Pain relievers
Over-the-counter (OTC) pain medications often help to minimize your discomfort, particularly at the start of the recovery period. Commonly used OTC pain relievers include aspirin, acetaminophen (Tylenol, others), ibuprofen (Advil, Motrin, others) and naproxen (Aleve, others). Long-term use of these medications typi-

cally isn't recommended because of the distressing side effects this may cause, such as gastrointestinal bleeding, stomach upset, dizziness, bloating and abdominal pain.

Stronger prescription medications, such as codeine, are available for severe pain but these may cause constipation, which can be particularly distressing if you have persistent back pain. Long-term use may also create a tolerance for these medications, requiring larger dosages to alleviate the pain.

Bed rest

Acute pain from a compression fracture will usually diminish with 2 to 3 days of bed rest. A firm mattress provides better support for your spine than does a soft one. Although rest is essential to alleviate the initial pain, staying in bed for more than a few days may weaken your back and aggravate bone loss. It's also important to start moving as soon as you can, alternating periods of rest with activity. Physical activity can strengthen the muscles in your back and abdomen and improve support for your spine.

Bracing

If pain persists following several days of bed rest, your doctor may recommend that you use a brace to support your back. These back supports are generally worn for short periods of time, for example, when you're involved in activities that may cause a strain. Wearing a brace for too long can actually be counterproductive because your back doesn't work to support itself and may weaken.

Back braces are available at pharmacies and medical supply stores. There are many types and styles of braces to choose from. They can even be custom fit. Your doctor can advise you on the best choice for you.

Exercise

Exercise can strengthen your back muscles, help maintain your posture, slow bone loss and improve your overall fitness, all of which can help prevent fractures. Your doctor or physical therapist can help you design a safe exercise routine that provides you with these benefits while minimizing the risk of fractures during exercise.

Exercises usually include:

Weight-bearing exercise. Activities you do on your feet with your bones supporting your weight, such as walking

Resistance exercise. Activities that apply force on specific muscles and bones, for example, through the use of weights

Back-strengthening exercise. Activities that help you maintain or improve your posture, which helps avoid more fractures

Always be sure to consult your doctor or physical therapist before beginning an exercise program, as some activities or movements can increase the pain from compression fractures or even cause more fractures.

Vertebroplasty

Vertebroplasty (ver-TEE-bro-plas-tee) is a surgical procedure that uses an X-ray-guided needle to inject acrylic bone cement into fractured and collapsed vertebrae. The cement hardens over a few hours, sealing and stabilizing the fractures and relieving pain. The procedure generally takes from 1 to 2 hours.

Candidates for this procedure are people who have persistently unstable vertebral fractures caused by osteoporosis or the presence of a bone tumor. You'll likely undergo several tests before having the procedure, including a bone scan or magnetic resonance imaging (MRI), to make sure vertebroplasty is right for you. The procedure is usually performed when other noninvasive methods of treatment aren't successful.

Reports indicate that vertebroplasty provides complete or significant pain relief in 67 percent to 100 percent of cases. Some people feel pain relief immediately after the procedure, and most are able to return to normal activities on the same day.

Short-term complications are relatively few. During the hardening process, the cement generates heat that threatens nerve endings within the spine. This may cause temporary discomfort, but may also provide some of the pain relief associated with vertebroplasty.

One of the main concerns surrounding vertebroplasty is leakage of the cement into surrounding tissues as it's being injected. During test studies, the leakage generally had no side effects, although in a few incidents it led to compressed nerves and increased pain.

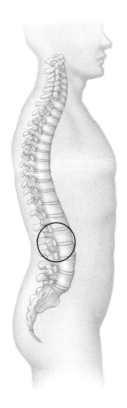

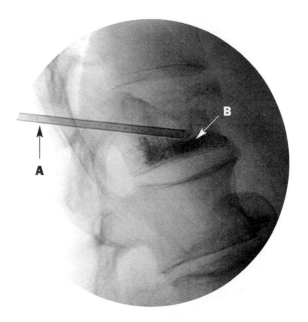

During the vertebroplasty procedure, a surgeon will view an X-ray image (above) in order to guide a needle (A) to a fractured vertebra. Bone cement injected into the vertebra (B) helps stabilize the fracture.

Although vertebroplasty is an exciting possibility for treating compression fractures, investigators emphasize that the procedure's short-term and long-term risks and benefits are still unclear. In particular, health experts question whether this procedure might cause vertebral fractures in the areas next to the repaired vertebra.

Kyphoplasty

A surgical procedure related to vertebroplasty is kyphoplasty (KI-fo-plas-tee), but kyphoplasty involves the use of a balloon-tipped needle. After the needle is inserted into the vertebra, the balloon is inflated to create a space for the cement to be injected. In most cases, this action not only strengthens the vertebra but also may expand the collapsed vertebral body.

Kyphoplasty provides a high incidence of pain relief, and serious complications are uncommon. But again, health experts caution that more research is necessary to ascertain all of the procedure's risks and benefits.

Treating hip fractures

Surgery is almost always the best way to repair a hip fracture. Doctors typically turn to nonsurgical alternatives, such as traction, only if you have a serious illness that makes surgery too risky. The type of surgery you have generally depends on where the bone is broken, the severity of the fracture and your age.

Femoral neck fractures

The long bone of your thigh (femur) is connected to the pelvis at your hip, which is a ball-and-socket joint. A narrow section of the femur just below the joint, known as the femoral neck, is a common location for a hip fracture. Doctors repair the fracture by one of three methods:

Internal fixation. If the broken bone is still properly aligned, the doctor may insert metal screws into the bone to hold it together while the fracture heals.

Partial femur replacement. If the ends of the broken bone aren't properly aligned or if they're damaged or shattered, the doctor may remove the head and neck of the femur and insert an artificial replacement, which is called a prosthesis (pros-THEE-sis). This surgical procedure is known as hemiarthroplasty (hem-e-AHR-thro-plas-tee).

Total hip replacement. This procedure involves replacing the entire upper femur with a prosthesis. Total hip replacement may be a good option if arthritis or a prior injury has damaged the joint, affecting its function before the fracture.

Intertrochanteric region fractures

The intertrochanteric region is the part of a femur adjacent to the femoral neck. To repair a fracture in this area, a surgeon usually inserts a long metal screw, known as a hip compression screw, through the fracture to rejoin the broken bone. The screw is attached to a plate that runs partially down the length of the femur. The plate is attached to the femur with smaller screws to keep the bone stable. As the bone heals, the compression screw allows the edges to grow together.

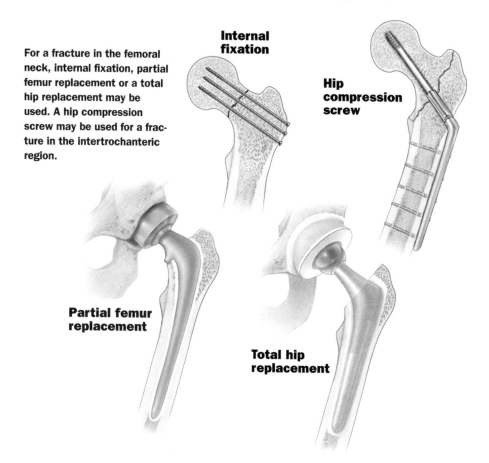

For a fracture in the femoral neck, internal fixation, partial femur replacement or a total hip replacement may be used. A hip compression screw may be used for a fracture in the intertrochanteric region.

Internal fixation

Hip compression screw

Partial femur replacement

Total hip replacement

General concerns about hip surgery

When you have hip surgery, you'll either undergo general anesthesia or local anesthesia. If all or part of the joint is removed, the prosthesis is often secured with bone cement — the same type that's used in vertebroplasty and kyphoplasty. It takes only a few hours for the cement to harden and the hip replacement to be firmly in place. Sometimes a different type of prosthesis is used that allows the bone itself to grow into the device and keep it in place. Receiving a cementless hip replacement usually requires a longer recovery period because the bone needs time to grow. A hybrid prosthesis involves cementing part of the device — usually the socket — and leaving the other part — usually the femoral neck — uncemented.

Artificial hip joints can function well for 20 years or more, but eventually the prosthesis may loosen, necessitating another operation. Older adults are more likely to receive a partial or total hip replacement, as they tend to put less strain on an artificial joint than younger people do. The internal fixation method is more common with younger people, but it can be used for fractures in people of any age so long as the broken bones are well aligned.

If the hip is infected or there's a skin disorder around the hip, a surgeon will likely wait until the conditions improve before doing the operation. Before surgery you'll probably go through an extensive evaluation to check your medical history, the extent of damage to your hip and the condition of your heart and lungs. Your doctor will also discuss the potential risks and benefits of hip surgery in your specific case.

At the hospital

Hip surgery usually requires a 3- to 10-day hospital stay, depending on how well you recover from the operation. At the hospital you'll be given medication to control postoperative pain. The hospital staff will also help you get moving as soon as possible.

A serious complication of hip surgery is the formation of blood clots in the veins of your thighs and calves. A blood clot may break free and travel to your lungs, causing a pulmonary embolism that can be fatal in a matter of hours. The hospital staff will closely monitor your condition to prevent this from happening.

It's important to begin gentle activity immediately after surgery. This may include slowly moving your foot up and down or rotating your ankle as you lie in bed. A physical therapist can also show you how to do specific exercises. Although these activities might feel uncomfortable at first, they can lessen pain, prevent blood clot formation and improve hip movement.

You'll continue these exercises after you go home. In addition, your doctor will likely prescribe blood-thinning medications for several weeks or months after the procedure to prevent clot formation, as well as antibiotics to prevent infections.

Some older adults, particularly those who live alone, temporarily enter a rehabilitation center after surgery to receive physical therapy and assistance during their recovery. Others may need permanent assistance.

At home

Before you go home, or even before you enter the hospital for surgery, it may be a good idea to have your living space rearranged to be more conducive to recovery. Clear pathways so that you can freely use a walker, and make sure that you have available a firm, high-seated chair. Set up a personal recovery center with everything you need at your fingertips, such as eyeglasses, reading material, medications, a phone, a remote control, tissues, a wastebasket and a drinking glass and pitcher.

You can contribute much to your own rehabilitation. Your participation in the recovery process often determines the procedure's success. Here are a number of factors to keep in mind:

- Keep the incision clean and dry. Stitches are generally removed 2 to 3 weeks after surgery. Until then take sponge baths instead of showers or full baths.
- Swelling is a normal reaction during the first 3 to 6 months after surgery. To counteract the swelling, elevate your leg and place an ice pack on your hip for several minutes at a time. Avoid placing ice directly on your skin by wrapping the pack in a washcloth or dish towel.
- Contact your doctor immediately if you think you're developing a blood clot or infection. Signs and symptoms of a blood clot include pain, redness or tenderness in your calf and new swelling in your leg or foot. Signs and symptoms of an infection include redness or swelling around the incision, wound drainage, persistent high fever, chills and increasing hip pain.
- Care must be taken not to dislocate the prosthesis. Don't cross your legs, whether sitting, standing or lying down. Keep your knees below the level of your hips. Sit on a cushion to keep your hips higher than your knees. Avoid bending at the waist. When sleeping, place a pillow between your knees to keep your hip properly aligned.
- Because bacteria often enter through your mouth during dental surgery, it's important to let your dentist know that you've had a hip replacement. Taking antibiotics before dental work can help prevent an infection. Take this precaution for the rest of your life.

Hip protectors

Wearing special padding may help prevent hip fractures. A recent study revealed that people who wore hip protectors — special undergarments designed to hold padded shields — were 60 percent less likely to break a hip than those who didn't wear them. If you think a hip protector might work for you, talk to your doctor. The protectors cost about $80 and are available at medical supply stores.

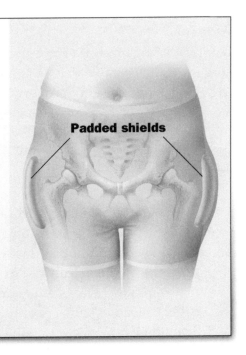

Padded shields

- It's always important to stay active. Get up and move around at least once for each hour during the day. If you have a cemented or hybrid prosthesis, you can usually put some weight on your leg right away, but you'll need to use a walker for 4 to 6 weeks to allow the joint to heal properly. If you have a cementless prosthesis, your surgeon will probably ask you not to put any weight on the leg for the first 6 weeks, to give your bones time to grow into the prosthesis.
- At the same time, don't overdo your activities. The key is to be active and exercise at a level that's comfortable for you. Walking is usually safe, and swimming, an exercise that's easy on your joints, is recommended after your incision has healed.
- A healthy diet is also important. If you were watching your weight before surgery, continue doing so because excess weight can place unnecessary stress on your hip joint.

Most people eventually return to their normal activities after hip surgery. But it doesn't happen immediately. A healthy recovery requires not only a willingness to do what your doctor or physical therapist prescribes but also consistency in actually following through on that advice.

Treating wrist fractures

Compared with vertebral and hip fractures, wrist fractures are usually much simpler to treat. Most osteoporotic wrist fractures — about 90 percent — are clean breaks of the radius bone in the forearm just above the wrist joint. This break is known as a Colles' fracture. Such fractures typically heal well, and full use of the hand and wrist is usually restored.

But some wrist fractures can be complex. If the broken ends of bone shift apart by less than a tenth of an inch (2 millimeters), the fracture is considered displaced, and the bone must be realigned before it's allowed to heal. If the bone splinters into numerous broken pieces, the break is called a comminuted (KOM-ih-NOOT-ud) fracture. In either case, surgery may be required to reposition the pieces and put in various devices to hold them in place as the bone heals. If broken bone breaks the skin — an open fracture — emergency treatment is required to prevent infection.

Your doctor may choose from several methods of treatment:

Cast or splint. A cast is often the preferred method for older adults who have a simple wrist fracture with minimal displacement. A short-arm cast is often applied from below the elbow to the hand. This immobilizes the wrist bone, is less invasive than surgery and usually has good results. After a fracture, swelling is often a problem. If so, a splint may be used for the first few days and then replaced with a cast after the swelling has subsided. Elevating your arm and icing your hand helps to diminish the swelling.

In other cases, a long-arm cast, which extends from your upper arm to your hand, is used to immobilize the whole arm and thumb. The long-arm cast is later replaced with a short-arm cast to allow free motion of the elbow. After the cast is removed, your doctor may have you use a removable splint at night and between exercise sessions during the day for added support.

External fixation. If a fracture is severely displaced or comminuted, it may heal best with metal pins inserted through the skin into the bone on either side of the fracture. The pins are attached externally to a frame to help hold the fracture in place. Your arm is held in a sling for elevation and protection. The device is usually

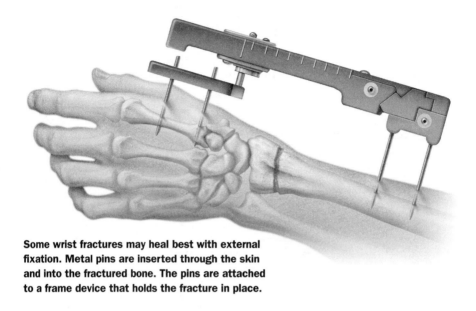

Some wrist fractures may heal best with external fixation. Metal pins are inserted through the skin and into the fractured bone. The pins are attached to a frame device that holds the fracture in place.

worn for 6 to 12 weeks. During this time the pins can be adjusted to ensure the precise alignment of the bone.

Internal fixation. Some complex fractures, particularly those that extend into the joint, may require internal fixation. During open surgery a surgeon may place metal pins, rods, plates or screws inside or along the fracture to hold the bone in position.

Percutaneous pins. *Percutaneous* (per-ku-TAY-ne-us) means "through the skin." With this procedure, freestanding metal or biodegradable pins or wires are inserted into the fractured area and maneuvered to align the bone fragments. A disadvantage of this method is that the pins often don't provide enough stability, especially in older adults. Thus, the technique may be combined with external fixation.

Injectable bone cement. Researchers are working on a new type of bone cement that hardens within minutes and stabilizes bone fragments in wrist or vertebral fractures. This cement is different from the acrylic cement currently used in vertebroplasty, kyphoplasty and some hip replacements. The new type is bioactive, which means that it's eventually resorbed into your body during the process of bone remodeling and replaced with natural bone. One type of bioactive cement is already approved by the Food and Drug Administration. Other formulations are also being developed.

Physical therapy. A frequent complication of a wrist fracture is the subsequent stiffness of the wrist. To counteract this effect, your doctor or physical therapist will work with you to get your fingers, elbow and shoulder moving as soon as possible after the fracture has stabilized. A common exercise is to close your fingers into a fist and then slowly and fully extend them. You may be asked to do this several times every hour during the day. After the cast or fixation device is removed, you'll be given additional exercises, including resistance exercises to build bone mass. You may also receive balance and gait training to prevent further falls.

As in any rehabilitation, you play a vital role. Keep in mind that your goal is to regain function of your hand, and you may accomplish this by following your doctor's instructions carefully and by consistently performing the prescribed exercises.

Managing chronic pain

Although proper treatment may relieve the initial hurt of an osteoporotic fracture, the recovery period following treatment also can be painful. Sometimes pain may persist after the bone has healed.

Dealing with chronic pain can be frustrating when there seems to be no immediate relief in sight. The pain can cause feelings of irritability, depression and anxiety, which only makes the physical pain seem worse. Although no quick fixes are available, you can do something to manage your pain. Start with two key concepts:
- You play a central role in pain management. If you want your life to improve, you'll need to take steps to make it happen. Only you can control your future.
- Managing chronic pain isn't about making pain disappear. It's about learning to keep pain at a level you can tolerate. It's about enjoying life again, despite the pain.

In dealing with chronic pain, people often turn to pain medications. These are certainly appropriate for coping with acute pain and can be very effective when used properly. But for many chronic pain problems, medication may not be the answer. Some people take medication because they feel they need to, not because it helps. The drugs become a crutch or distraction from more effective, safer, long-term solutions. These people are often surprised to find that stopping their medication isn't as difficult as they had anticipated. They also often find that not using drugs gives them a greater sense of control over the pain and their life.

So what are the alternatives to pain medication? Here are a number of options:

Exercise. Although rest is important for recovery and pain relief, exercise is equally vital to reducing pain, especially in the long term. Exercise causes your body to release chemicals called endorphins which block pain signals from reaching your brain. The more endorphins you produce on your own, the less you need to rely on other forms of pain management, such as medication.

Because certain exercises shouldn't be done when you have osteoporosis, it's important to consult your doctor before beginning exercise. That way you'll be sure you're performing the activities that are best for you.

Ice and heat. Applying an ice pack can reduce swelling and inflammation and act as a local anesthetic. Treatment in the form of a hot water bottle, hot bath or heat lamp relaxes your muscles and helps relieve chronic pain. Remember not to directly expose your skin to extreme temperatures. Keep the ice pack or hot water bottle wrapped in a towel. Limit applications to 20 minutes at a time.

Relaxation techniques. Your physical therapist can show you certain relaxation techniques that help take your mind off pain, relax your muscles and relieve unnecessary stress. Such techniques might include visualization, progressive muscle relaxation and deep breathing.

Biofeedback. The goal of biofeedback is to teach you how to control certain body responses. During a biofeedback session, a trained therapist applies electrodes and other sensors to various parts of your body. The electrodes are attached to devices that monitor your responses and give you visual or auditory feedback of your muscle tension, heart rate, blood pressure, breathing rate and skin temperature.

With this feedback you can learn to produce positive changes in body functions, such as lowering your blood pressure or raising

Set SMART goals

When you're in pain, it's easy for the discomfort to become the center of your attention. Other things in life that were once important to you may take a back seat to the pain.

Setting goals helps divert your attention from chronic pain and provides an opportunity to think about your lifestyle and what you can do to better manage your pain. But goal setting isn't as easy as it sounds. You simply can't identify a couple of things you want and expect them to happen. You'll only be setting yourself up for disappointment. Set goals that are SMART — that is, goals that are specific, measurable, attainable, realistic and trackable. Here's how:

- **Specific.** State exactly what you want to achieve and how you're going to do it. Set goals that you can achieve within a week to a month. It's easy to give up on goals that take too long to reach. Break down a large goal into a series of smaller weekly or daily goals. After you achieve one of the smaller goals, move on to the next.
- **Measurable.** A goal doesn't do you any good if there's no way of telling if you've achieved it. "I want to feel better" isn't a good goal. It's variable. "I want to work 8 hours each day" is a good goal. It's specific and it's measurable.
- **Attainable.** Ask yourself if a goal is within reasonable reach. Completing a power-walking marathon may not be an achievable goal if your previous exercising was limited. But scheduling several brisk walks daily may be attainable.
- **Realistic.** Goal setting helps take your focus off pain and onto your future. But you can't ignore your limitations. Your goals need to be within your capabilities. If you've suffered a serious back injury, a goal of returning to a job that involves heavy lifting may not be realistic. Instead, your goal might be a job in a related field or going back to school for retraining.
- **Trackable.** Being able to track your progress encourages you to keep going and reach your goal. Look for ways to chart your improvements.

your skin temperature. These are signs of relaxation. The biofeed-back therapist may use relaxation techniques to further calm you.

Electrical stimulation. Transcutaneous electrical nerve stimulation (TENS) may help stop pain by blocking nerve signals from reaching your brain. A physical therapist places electrodes on your skin near the area of your pain. TENS may relieve pain in your leg due to inflammation or compression of nerves in your back, but it may provide little relief for chronic back pain.

A word of caution. Certain methods of pain relief may spell trouble if you have osteoporosis. Massage, chiropractic treatment and other spinal manipulation can cause or aggravate vertebral fractures, so talk to your doctor before trying any of these.

Chapter 13

Home safety

Falls are a serious hazard for older adults, especially those with low bone density or osteoporosis. Here are some sobering statistics. According to the Centers for Disease Control and Prevention, one out of every three people 65 years and older in the United States will fall each year. And of those who fall, 20 percent to 30 percent will suffer moderate to severe injuries that reduce their mobility and independence. At least 95 percent of all hip fractures result from a fall.

Also, did you know that for people age 65 and older, half of all falls occur at home? It's simple logic that a part of any action plan for osteoporosis involves minimizing your risk of falling. You may do so by organizing your home environment and work space in a way that allows you to function and move about comfortably and safely.

You may also have occasion to use what are known as assistive devices. These are items or pieces of equipment that enable you to perform routine tasks and activities safely and with minimum stress. Canes and walkers can provide support and keep you balanced as you move about. Other assistive devices eliminate dangerous movements that can lead to fracture, such as reaching above your head for something on a high shelf or bending forward to pick up something off the floor.

If you're like most people, you probably want your life to remain independent. Often, this means being able to live at home, keeping your own schedule and organizing your time as freely as anyone else does. To be able to do this for as long a time as reasonably possible, some preventive action is necessary. This chapter focuses on practical measures you can take to help you prevent fractures, stay active and maintain the lifestyle you want.

Staying safe indoors

It's ironic that the home — your private sanctum, your safety net — ranks statistically as one of the most dangerous places you can be. But you have to remember that the average residence puts you in regular contact with electricity, heat sources, water, slick surfaces, stairs and a multitude of other physical dangers. And many people, particularly older adults, spend a major portion of each 24-hour day within the walls of their homes.

For those reasons, it's important to survey your home with your own safety in mind. Look for features that could cause you to lose your balance or footing: stairs, rugs, electrical cords, step stools and locations in the home where there may be wet surfaces. The kitchen and bathroom are often among the most dangerous places in the home. Also identify high-traffic areas that combine multiple threats.

Keep in mind these general principles when inspecting your home for safety: Keep pathways clear, use proper lighting and safe seating, and organize work areas.

Keep pathways clear

Clearly, you need to watch your footing everywhere you go in your home. But pay close attention to the primary pathways within rooms, between rooms and in hallways. Keep these areas picked up and remove unnecessary clutter. Be alert to tight spaces and blind corners that might cause you to bump into furniture or collide with someone. Avoid loose rugs and carpeting, buckled or torn linoleum or tile, and raised thresholds — the crosspiece at the bottom of a door frame — that could catch your heel and cause a fall.

Taking steps to prevent falls

Here are some common-sense changes you can make inside your home to help prevent falls:

- Keep rooms free of clutter, especially floors.
- Keep electrical and telephone cords tucked out of the way.
- Avoid walking in socks, stockings or plush slippers. Choose comfortable, low-heeled shoes with nonskid soles.
- Be sure your carpets and rugs have skidproof backing or are tacked to the floor. Get rid of throw rugs.
- Place a phone and flashlight within reach of your bed.
- Make sure stairs are well lit and have handrails on both sides. Cover the steps with tightly woven carpet or nonslip treads.
- Install grab bars on bathroom walls near the tub, shower and toilet. Use a rubber mat in the tub and shower.
- Use a night light in your bathroom.
- Add ceiling fixtures so that you don't have to walk into a dark room to turn on a lamp.

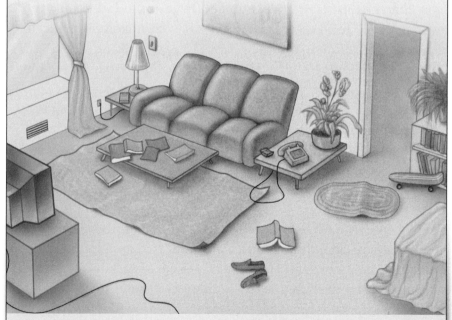

There are at least 13 hazards that cause falls in this illustration. Can you find them?

Answers on page 189.

Use proper lighting

Good vision is one of the best tools you have to prevent falls. The easiest, most practical way to improve vision safety in your home is to add lighting. Be prepared to add more than just an extra lamp or two. Start by increasing the wattage in the lamps you currently use. Be careful to stay within the manufacturers' recommended range for each fixture, which is marked on the device.

Consider a combination of incandescent, fluorescent and halogen lighting. Fluorescent bulbs usually produce fewer shadows. Incandescent lamps provide greater contrast, and halogen lighting is thought to come closest to sunlight. Be aware, also, that too much light used in the wrong way can produce a blinding glare.

Areas of your home that may need the greatest lighting improvement are stairways, hallways, storage closets, storage sheds, the laundry room, the garage and locations with a change in floor height, for example, a sunken living room.

Ask an electrician about adding three- or four-way wall switches to your heavily used rooms. These allow you to control lights from more than one location, saving you a trip across a dark room. The technology for remote control switches has improved dramatically, as has the cost of these safety devices.

Your balance may not be as good in the dark as it is during daylight hours. Place night lights in key pathways of your house. They're great for illuminating midnight trips to the bathroom and kitchen. Check to see that you have the highest-wattage bulbs allowed in overhead lights. Installing fluorescent lighting under kitchen cabinets helps light work areas.

Use safe seating

Keep furniture, especially chairs, sofas and other forms of seating, in good repair. Chairs should be well supported and not prone to tipping. Be cautious with anything on rollers or rockers. To prevent dizziness that contributes to falls, sit down or stand up slowly.

It's important that seating allow you to sit down or stand up easily and without unnecessary strain. Particularly after hip replacement, you'll need to keep your hips higher than your knees to prevent dislocating the new joint. Chairs or sofas that sit high

> **Hazards from page 187**
> 1. Skateboard near door, 2. Bookshelf near door, 3. Throw rug near door, 4. Books on floor, 5. Slippers in pathway, 6. Telephone cord, 7. Raised carpet edges, 8. TV cord in walkway, 9. Low coffee table, 10. Low table near door, 11. Long tablecloth end, 12. Long window curtain, 13. Deep sofa that's difficult to sit down in or get out of

with firm cushioning are generally easier to get in and out of than low, soft-cushioned seating. You may be able to adapt existing furniture with an extra foam cushion or two placed on the chair or under the sofa cushioning.

Organize work areas

Keep frequently used items within easy reach and avoid stretching for items on high shelves. If you must retrieve something high above you, use a sturdy step stool with wide steps and handrails or an assistive device known as a reacher. In the kitchen you can limit strain on your back by using front burners on your stove whenever possible and sliding, not lifting, pots in and out of the oven. Clean up any spills on the floor immediately. Exposure to tap water that's too hot can cause you to pull back suddenly and possibly slip and fall, especially in the bathtub. To prevent scalding from hot water, be sure the water heater thermostat isn't set too high.

Assistive devices: Help around the house

Everyone has heard the phrase, "Work smarter, not harder." If you swap the word "live" for "work," you'll begin to understand the idea behind assistive devices. These tools for living smarter can help you with everyday tasks. Some are simple handle extensions that provide more leverage, and others are sophisticated, ergonomically designed devices.

Gadgets and gimcracks aren't for you, you say? That initial reaction is typical — even understandable. But before you associate assistive devices with wasted money or physical weakness, consider how many of them we already rely on to make our lives easier and more enjoyable.

It's unlikely, for example, that you hesitate before climbing into an automobile for a short drive to the grocery store. A car is an assistive device. The vehicle certainly helps you get from one point to another with greater speed and comfort than you would have by walking. What about the remote control that allows you to flick through television channels while seated in a comfortable chair across the room? A remote control also is an assistive device.

Assistive devices generally have a well-defined function and are easy to use, sometimes with a little practice. Whether it's something you do every day, such as putting on your shoes, or once in a while, like moving a heavy object, these aids help you achieve your goals with minimum risk to your bones. Gait aids, such as a cane or walker, allow you to put more energy into mobility and less into stability — you can walk farther, faster and more safely.

Medical supply stores, Web sites, catalogs, your hospital's physical therapy department and even the local hardware store are full of specifically designed items and materials that can help you with daily tasks. By using these tools, you can ease pain, add comfort, increase safety, bolster confidence, enhance ability and sustain independence.

Devices for daily needs

Assistive devices are often used to accomplish simple daily tasks. Using the right tool can facilitate almost everything you need to do or want to do at home. One of the most common and practical tools is what's known as a reacher. This device is a lightweight pole with a trigger at one end that manipulates a single grasping claw at the other end. A reacher can help you retrieve lightweight items such as a newspaper from the floor or a remote control from the coffee table without having to bend forward. The device is easily carried and can be used just about anywhere in the house.

Many such helpful devices are available for use in the bathroom. These include grab bars and folding shower seats to prevent slipping, and elevated toilets that permit easier seating. You can buy long-handled hairbrushes, combs and sponges to clean and groom yourself without having to twist or bend your torso.

In the kitchen, chances are you're already using some small electric appliances. You can expand their usefulness by finding new ways to adapt them to your chores. Manufacturers of appliances sometimes include tips for alternative uses. Buy a jar opener that can be mounted under a kitchen cabinet or countertop. A reacher with a squeeze-handle grasper is perfect for easy access to items on higher or lower shelves.

Devices for movement and mobility

If you've had hip surgery, it's likely you'll need support as you move around the house, at least during the months of recovery. Multiple compression fractures of the spine that cause you to hunch forward also may require you to use a cane or walker. According to the Department of Health and Human Services, more than 7 million Americans use assistive devices to accommodate impairments with walking. Although they may at first seem awkward and annoying, walking aids actually increase your independence by helping you get around on your own.

Walking aids include canes and walkers. Each type comes in a variety of sizes, weights and designs, so it's not always easy to select and properly use the right one. It may be best to have your doctor or physical therapist recommend something that would be most appropriate for you. The same individual can help you determine the proper size and fit, as well as the best way to use it and adapt it to your needs.

It's a common mistake to choose a cane that's too long. The extra length pushes up one arm and shoulder, causing strain to those muscles and to the back. Awkwardness with any new device is natural. Remember the first time you tried riding a bike or casting a fishing rod? Ease will come with practice. Here are some pointers to help you be more informed about your options.

Canes

Canes are not intended to carry the full weight of your body. Rather, they provide some relief and stability by allowing you to put a third point of contact on the ground (besides your two feet). If you need to use your cane daily, the traditional J-handle (candy-cane) style may not be your best choice. That's because with a J-handle your weight isn't centered over the cane's shaft, which puts more pressure on your hand. Instead, consider using the swan-neck cane, in which the shaft absorbs more of your weight. Other hand-grip styles and shapes are available. Choose the one that feels most comfortable. Quadripod canes, which have four feet, offer greater stability than canes with a single tip but can be cumbersome to use. A lightweight aluminum cane is often less of a burden than a heavier wooden one.

To see if your cane is the right fit, stand erect with your shoes on, letting your arms hang at your sides. The top of the cane's handle should align with the crease of your wrist. When you hold the cane while standing still, your elbow should be flexed at a 15- to 20-degree angle. Wooden canes must be cut to the correct height. Adjustable canes can be lengthened or shortened to fit.

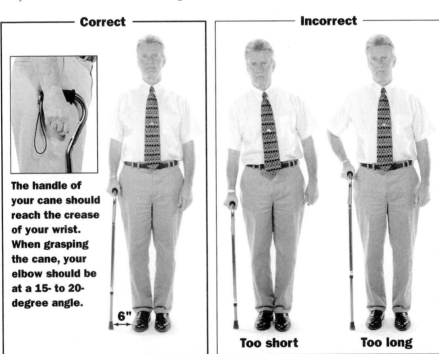

Correct — **Incorrect**

The handle of your cane should reach the crease of your wrist. When grasping the cane, your elbow should be at a 15- to 20-degree angle.

6"

Too short   **Too long**

A proper fit for your cane is important. Canes that are the wrong height for you can cause falls as well as arm and back pain.

It's best to hold your cane in the hand opposite the side that needs support, regardless of which hand is your dominant or preferred hand. The cane and the affected leg should swing forward and touch the ground at the same time. On stairs, step up with your good leg, then bring your injured leg and cane up. This way, your good leg lifts your body. Coming down the stairs, lead with your injured leg and cane, then bring your good leg down. This allows your good leg to lower your body.

Walkers

Walkers are self-standing and provide more stability than does a cane. Some are maneuvered by lifting, and others are equipped with wheels. They often have a basket or carrying case. Walkers function best in single-level homes and shouldn't be used on stairs or in crowded, cluttered areas.

In general, walkers with wheels are easier to manage than walkers that you lift, unless you have thick carpet or are on rough ground. Wheeled walkers are especially important to use if you have balance problems. If you'll be doing any traveling, consider a walker that folds.

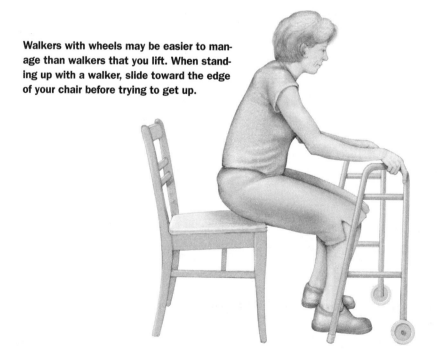

Walkers with wheels may be easier to manage than walkers that you lift. When standing up with a walker, slide toward the edge of your chair before trying to get up.

As with a cane, walkers need to be adjusted to the correct height. When your arms are relaxed at your sides, the top of the walker should align with the crease in your wrist. If your walker is adjusted correctly, you should be able to stand up straight when using it.

Because a walker disrupts your normal walking gait, you'll need a little practice. To walk, move the walker a comfortable arm's length from you. Don't move it too far in front or you might fall. Then step into the walker, leading with your weak or injured leg. Don't attempt to climb stairs or use an escalator with a walker unless you have had specific training to do this.

Grips and tips

On any walking aid, a handle contoured to your grip is usually easier to hold for extended periods than a rounded handle. Wrap foam around a handle that feels too small.

The tips of walking devices come in different diameters and styles. What's important is the traction they provide with the ground. Rubber is a commonly used material because it's nonskid and easily replaced when worn out. Flat, soft tips hold the ground more securely than rounded ones do. Never glue on tips. You'll need to replace them as they wear out. Most pharmacies and some hardware stores carry replacement tips.

Take your time

If you're going to be using a walking aid for a while, invest some time in choosing the right style and fit for you. You can find walking aids at medical supply stores and some pharmacies. You can also order them from specialty catalogs or online.

As for cost, more expensive models aren't necessarily better at providing support than less expensive ones are. Medicare or your private insurance company may cover part or all of the cost of your walking aid if you have a written prescription from your doctor.

An open mind

Assistive devices can't do all things for all people. You can't expect a single implement to free you from all the problems you face from osteoporosis or allow you to be totally independent. But assistive devices can still have a tremendous impact. It's common for people to marvel over how much easier life has become with that extra little bit of assistance, once they start using them. To maintain your independence, keep an open mind about your physical limitations — a realistic grasp of what you can and can't do — and the tools that can help you overcome or minimize these limitations.

Whether you use assistive devices depends on you and your doctor or occupational therapist. Some of the tools described in this chapter may or may not be right for you. For a more customized evaluation, contact an occupational therapist. Occupational therapists specialize in helping people deal with the effects of illness, injury or aging in their daily life. A therapist typically can meet with you on an individual basis and make recommendations based on your specific needs. Assistive devices can be obtained from a hospital's physical therapy department, medical supply stores, specialized catalogs or Internet sites, and even local hardware stores.

The importance of attitude

All this talk about prevention and assistive devices and safe movements may leave you feeling as if life has definitely changed, and not for the better. What happened to the days when you moved around and did whatever you pleased without giving it a second thought? Though the following may sound cliched, it still rings true: One of the constant things in life is change. How you cope with change can have a big impact on your quality of life.

Your attitude toward osteoporosis and the adjusted lifestyle it may entail makes a tremendous difference in how independent or dependent you eventually become. For example, if you look at your cane as a sign of weakness and deterioration in your body, you might avoid using it and end up falling and breaking a hip. But if you view your cane as a symbol of freedom and opportunity, you'll make it work for you. You'll benefit from the support and stability it provides, and you'll value the ability to move around without the aid of others.

Taking control

It's never too late to work on maintaining or improving bone health. This book discusses many ways to approach this. A well-organized action plan suited to your needs and abilities allows you to benefit from diet, exercise, medications, good posture, and a safe environment at home or work. Just as important to success is the support you receive from your doctor, other health care professionals and your family and friends. All of these factors in combination can provide you with the means to prevent or treat osteoporosis and maintain a full and active life.

Additional resources

Contact these organizations for more information about osteoporosis, good bone health and various factors of your osteoporosis action plan, such as diet, exercise and home safety.

Administration on Aging (AOA)

U. S. Department of Health and Human Services
200 Independence Ave. S.W.
Washington, DC 20201
(202) 619-0724
www.aoa.dhhs.gov

American Academy of Orthopaedic Surgeons

6300 N. River Road
Rosemont, IL 60018-4262
(847) 823-7186 or (800) 346-2267
www.aaos.org

American Academy of Physical Medicine and Rehabilitation

One IBM Plaza, Suite 2500
Chicago, IL 60611
(312) 464-9700
www.aapmr.org

American Association of Clinical Endocrinologists

1000 Riverside Ave., Suite 205
Jacksonville, FL 32204
(904) 353-7878
www.aace.com

American Dietetic Association

120 South Riverside Plaza, Suite 2000
Chicago, IL 60606-6995
(312) 899-0040 or (800) 877-1600
www.eatright.org

American Physical Therapy Association

1111 North Fairfax Street
Alexandria, VA 22314
(703) 684-2782 or (800) 999-2782
www.apta.org

Food and Drug Administration

5600 Fishers Lane
Rockville, MD 20857
(301) 827-4573 or (888) 463-6332
www.fda.gov

Food and Nutrition Information Center

National Agricultural Library, Room 105
10301 Baltimore Avenue
Beltsville, MD 20705
(301) 504-5719
www.nal.usda.gov/fnic

International Osteoporosis Foundation

71, cours Albert-Thomas
69447 Lyon Cedex 03
France
33-472-91-41-77
www.osteofound.org

Mayo Clinic Health Information

www.MayoClinic.com

National Center for Injury Prevention and Control

Mailstop K65
4770 Buford Highway N.E.
Atlanta, GA 30341
(770) 488-1506
www.cdc.gov/ncipc/ncipchm.htm

National Institute for Occupational Safety and Health

Education and Information Division
4676 Columbia Parkway, MSC 13
Cincinnati, OH 45226
(513) 533-8466 or (800) 356-4674
www.cdc.gov/niosh

National Institute of Arthritis and Musculoskeletal and Skin Diseases

National Institutes of Health
Building 31, Room 4C05
31 Center Drive, MSC 2350
Bethesda, MD 20892-2350
(301) 496-8190 or (877) 226-4267
www.niams.nih.gov

National Institute on Aging

National Institutes of Health
Building 31, Room 5C27
31 Center Drive, MSC 2292
Bethesda, MD 20892
(301) 496-1752
www.nia.nih.gov

National Osteoporosis Foundation

1232 22d St. N.W.
Washington, DC 20037-1292
(202) 223-2226 or (800) 223-9994
www.nof.org

National Rehabilitation Information Center

4200 Forbes Blvd., Suite 202
Lanham, MD 20706
(301) 459-5900 or (800) 346-2742
www.naric.com

National Safety Council

1121 Spring Lake Drive
Itasca, IL 60143
(630) 285-1121
www.nsc.org

National Women's Health Information Center

8550 Arlington Blvd., Suite 300
Fairfax, VA 22301
(703) 560-6618 or (800) 994-9662
www.4woman.org

National Women's Health Resource Center

120 Albany Street, Suite 820
New Brunswick, NJ 08901
(877) 986-9472
www.healthywomen.org

The North American Menopause Society

P. O. Box 94527
Cleveland, OH 44101
(440) 442-7550
www.menopause.org

North American Spine Society

22 Calendar Court, 2d Floor
LaGrange, IL 60525
(877) 774-6337
www.spine.org

Osteoporosis and Related Bone Diseases National Resource Center

National Institutes of Health
1232 22nd St. N.W.
Washington, DC 20037-1292
(202) 223-0344 or (800) 624-2663
www.osteo.org

Index

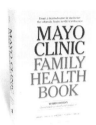

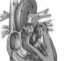

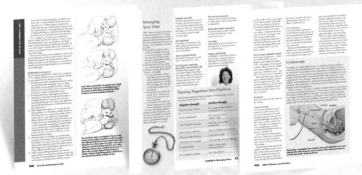

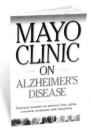

Mayo Clinic on Alzheimer's Disease
Practical answers on memory loss, aging, research, treatment and caregiving
Product # 270700 • $16.95

Alzheimer's disease robs you of your ability to think, reason and remember. This informative book provides concise, easy-to-understand information on the possible causes and treatments of Alzheimer's disease. Also included is the detailed section "A Quick Guide for Caregivers," a special reference for those caring for people with Alzheimer's disease. Includes diagrams, index and glossary.

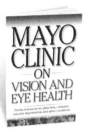

Mayo Clinic on Vision and Eye Health
Practical answers on glaucoma, cataracts, macular degeneration and other conditions
Product # 270600 • $14.95

Now learn the latest options from Mayo Clinic on preserving your precious vision and protecting the health of your eyes. *Mayo Clinic on Vision and Eye Health* offers scores of tips and ideas that you and your eye care professional can use to enhance your eye health.

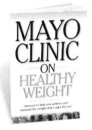

Mayo Clinic on Healthy Weight
Answers to help you achieve and maintain the weight that's right for you
Product # 270200 • $14.95

Featuring the Mayo Clinic Healthy Weight Pyramid developed by Mayo Clinic physicians and dietitians and based on research studies and practical experience. To help you achieve and maintain a healthy weight, this book explains the five steps to healthy eating and addresses proper nutrition, exercise and other factors affecting weight. Includes a four-color insert with charts and sample menus.

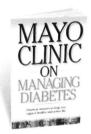

Mayo Clinic on Managing Diabetes
Practical answers to help you enjoy a healthy and active life
Product # 270300 • $14.95

This book provides practical knowledge and self-care advice to people with diabetes, so they can control their disease and lead healthy lives. Inside you'll find discussions on the underlying causes of diabetes and why achieving near-normal blood sugar values is important. It offers insight on how to monitor, manage and live with diabetes, along with information on how to prevent serious complications from the disease.

Order by calling 877-647-6397 and mention order code 180.
Or order online at *www.Healthe-store.com.*
Price does not include shipping and handling and applicable sales tax. All prices subject to change.

Mayo Clinic books are available at local bookstores.
When you purchase a Mayo Clinic publication, proceeds are used to further education and medical research at Mayo Clinic. You not only get answers to your questions, you become part of the solution.

When reliable information is what you need.

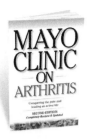

Mayo Clinic on Arthritis, Second Edition
Conquering the pain and leading an active life
Product # 268502 • $16.95

Arthritis can be disabling, but it doesn't have to defeat you. You can take control of your arthritis with the new information in *Mayo Clinic on Arthritis,* Second Edition. This new edition contains the best information we know to help you control your arthritis so that it doesn't control you.

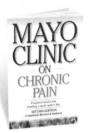

Mayo Clinic on High Blood Pressure, Second Edition
Taking charge of your hypertension
Product # 268402 • $16.95

High blood pressure is a very serious condition. By using the information in *Mayo Clinic on High Blood Pressure,* Second Edition, every day, you can live longer and better with high blood pressure, or help prevent it if you're at risk.

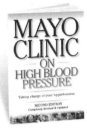

Mayo Clinic on Chronic Pain, Second Edition
Practical advice for leading a more active life
Product # 268702 • $16.95

Step by step, this brand-new edition of *Mayo Clinic on Chronic Pain* helps you regain control over your underlying condition as well as your daily symptoms. Mayo Clinic's experience with thousands of patients confirms that these techniques work. This easy-to-use book provides the specifics you need to take charge of your chronic pain and live a more active, productive and comfortable life.

Other Mayo Clinic books include:	*Product #*	*Price*
• Mayo Clinic Guide to Self-Care	270150	$22.95
• Mayo Clinic Heart Book, Second Edition	268150	$29.95
• Mayo Clinic on Depression	270500	$14.95
• Mayo Clinic on Digestive Health	268900	$14.95
• Mayo Clinic on Healthy Aging	270400	$14.95
• Mayo Clinic on Prostate Health, Second Edition	268803	$16.95

Health *e* Store

Order by calling 877-647-6397 and mention order code 180.
Or order online at *www.Healthe-store.com.*
Price does not include shipping and handling and applicable sales tax. All prices subject to change.

Mayo Clinic books are available at local bookstores.
When you purchase a Mayo Clinic publication, proceeds are used to further education and medical research at Mayo Clinic. You not only get answers to your questions, you become part of the solution.

MayoClinic.com

For additional information regarding your health and well-being, visit our Web site, MayoClinic.com, at *www.MayoClinic.com*. In the ever-changing health care environment, MayoClinic.com can provide you with continually updated information about healthy living and disease as well as advances in diagnosis and treatment.

MayoClinic.com is a trusted source for health information whether you have a newly diagnosed condition, face a major treatment decision or simply need a healthy recipe for dinner.

As in this book, MayoClinic.com provides trustworthy, practical and easy-to-understand information to help you live well and take charge of your health.

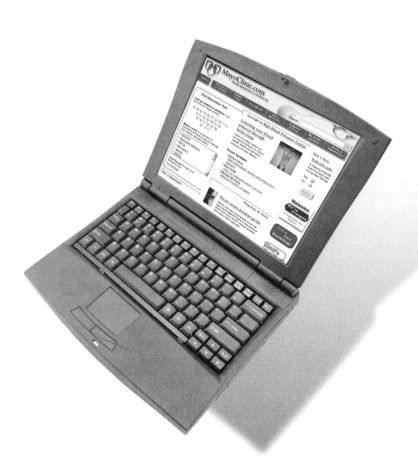

Reliable information for a healthier life.